Recent Results in Cancer Research

Fortschritte der Krebsforschung

Progrès dans les recherches sur le cancer

44

Edited by

Editor in chief
P. Rentchnick, Genève

Special Topics in Carcinogenesis

Edited by

E. Grundmann

With 54 Figures

Springer-Verlag Berlin · Heidelberg · New York 1974

Symposium of the "Gesellschaft zur Bekämpfung der Krebskrankheiten Nordrhein-Westfalen, e. V." Düsseldorf, 24th—25th March, 1972

Sponsored by the Swiss League against Cancer

ISBN-13: 978-3-642-80788-6 e-ISBN-13: 978-3-642-80786-2
DOI: 10.1007/978-3-642-80786-2

CONTENTS

Models of Experimental Carcinogenesis

List of Participants

Bannasch, P., Dr., Pathologisches Institut der Universität, D 8700 Würzburg, Luitpoldkrankenhaus

Chomette, G., M.D., Service d'Anatomie Pathologique, Groupe Hospitalier Pitié-Salpêtrière, 83 Bd. de l'Hospital, F Paris 13 E

Georgii, A., Dr., Pathologisches Institut der Medizinischen Hochschule, D 3000 Hannover-Kleefeld, Roderbruchstr. 101

Grundmann, E., Professor Dr., Pathologisches Institut der Universität, D 4400 Münster, Westring 17

Hamperl, H., Dr., Pathologisches Institut der Universität, D 5300 Bonn, Postfach

von der Helm, K., M.D., University of California, Department of Molecular Biology, Berkeley, CA 94720/USA

Hilfrich, J., Dr., Medizinische Hochschule Hannover, Abt. für experimentelle Pathologie, Theoretische Institute I, D 3000 Hannover-Kleefeld, Roderbruchstr. 101

Ivankovic, S., Dr., Deutsches Krebsforschungszentrum, Institut für experimentelle Toxikologie und Chemotherapie, D 6900 Heidelberg, Kirschnerstr. 6

Koss, L. G., M.D., Professor and Chairman, Department of Pathology, Albert Einstein College of Medicine at Montefiore Hospital and Medical Center, 111 East 210th Street, Bronx, NY 10467/USA

Laumonier, R., M.D., Faculté Mixte de Médicine et de Pharmacie, Hotel-Dieu, F 76 Rouen

Magee, P. N., M.D., Courtauld Institute of Biochemistry, The Middlesex Hospital, London W1P 5PR/Great Britain

Mennel, H. D., Dr., Max-Planck-Institut für Hirnforschung, Abt. für Allgemeine Neurologie, D 5000 Köln-Merheim, Ostmerheimer Str. 200

Mohr, U., Dr., Medizinische Hochschule Hannover, Abt. für experimentelle Pathologie, D 3000 Hannover-Kleefeld, Roderbruchstr. 101

Morris, H. P., M.D., Howard University, Research Professor of Biochemistry, Cancer Research Unit, Washington, D.C. 20001/USA

Munk, K., Dr., Deutsches Krebsforschungszentrum, Direktor, Institut für Virusforschung, D 6900 Heidelberg, Kirschnerstr. 6

NETTESHEIM, P., M.D., Oak Ridge National Laboratory, Post Office Box, Oak Ridge, TN 37830/USA

PONTÉN, J., M.D., Institut of Pathology, University, Uppsala/Schweden

PREUSSMANN, R., Dr., Deutsches Krebsforschungszentrum, Institut für experimentelle Geschwulsterzeugung und -behandlung, D 6900 Heidelberg, Berliner Str. 27

SANDBERG, A. A., M.D., Chief of Medicine C, Roswell Park Memorial Institute Department of Health, 666 Elm Street, Buffalo, NY 14203/USA

SCHREIBER, H., M.D., Oak Ridge National Laboratory, Post office Box Y, Oak Ridge, TN 37830/USA

SCHULZ, H., Dr., Chefarzt des Pathologischen Institutes, D 4500 Osnabrück, Natruper-Tor-Wall 1

STRÄULI, P., Dr., Institut für pathologische Anatomie der Universität, Abteilung Krebsforschung, Kantonspital Zürich, Schmelzbergstr. 12, CH 8006 Zürich

SUGANO, H., M.D., Cancer Institute, Toshima-ku, Tokyo/Japan

THOMAS, C., Dr., Pathologisches Institut der Universität, D 7800 Freiburg, Albertstraße 19

WIEBECKE, B., Dr., Pathologisches Institut der Universität, D 8000 München 15, Thalkirchnerstr. 36

WILLIGHAGEN, R. G. J., M.D., Pathologisch Laboratorium der Rijksuniversiteit te Leiden, Wassenaarseweg 62, Leiden/Holland

WOOD, S., M.D., Merck-Institute, Department of Experimental Pathology, Director, Rahway, NJ 07065/USA

WRBA, H., Dr., Institut für Krebsforschung der Universität, A 1090 Wien, IX, Borschkegasse 8 a

YOSIDA, T. H., National Institute of Genetics, Yata 1, Misima, Sizuoka-Ken/411 Japan

Welcome and Introduction

E. GRUNDMANN

On behalf of the "Gesellschaft zur Bekämpfung der Krebskrankheiten Nordrhein-Westfalen e. V." I welcome you in Düsseldorf. During these two days problems of oncogenesis have to be discussed. The participants have been selected with the intention of giving a review of the various fields which have some bearing on this topic. So you see here biochemists, cytologists, pathologists, immunologists, pharmacologists, virologists, and so on. Only by extensive cooperation of all scientists concerned in this field can this difficult problem of carcinogenesis ever be cleared up. Once the causal relations have been identified, we may have a reliable basis for cancer treatment.

Research on oncogenesis is of great interest, but it is only a part of the worldwide cancer campaign. It is our hope that this symposium will contribute towards helping the cancer patient. He is the center of all our efforts.

Keeping this in mind — let us begin!

Molecular Mechanisms in Chemical Carcinogenesis

P. N. MAGEE

Covalent binding of metabolites of the hepatocarcinogenic azo dye *p*-dimethylaminoazobenzene (DAB) to proteins of the livers of rats to which it had been administered was observed by JAMES and ELIZABETH MILLER in 1947. Since then a large amount of work on the interaction of many other chemical carcinogens with cellular macromolecules has been reported. It is now well established that most, perhaps all, chemical carcinogens become metabolically activated in the animal or are themselves chemically reactive and that various of the activated forms interact with tissue components *in vivo*. The terms precarcinogen, proximate carcinogen and ultimate carcinogen have been introduced by the MILLERS to describe the original, probably carcinogenically inactive compound, various intermediate metabolites of the carcinogen with greater carcinogenic activity and the final active carcinogenic form which is postulated to react at some crucial intracellular site and thus, in some as yet unknown manner, cause a normal cell to become a malignant one. It appears that, in general, the active forms of the chemical carcinogens are electrophilic reactants which react with nucleophilic centres in the cell (MILLER, E. C. and MILLER, J. A., 1966; MILLER, J. A., 1970; MILLER, J. A. and MILLER, E. C., 1966, 1971). Examples of such metabolic activations are the N-hydroxylation of aromatic amines and azo dyes, followed by esterification (MILLER, 1970) and the reduction of 4-nitroquinoline-N-oxide to 4-hydroxyaminoquinoline N-oxide (MATSUSHIMA and SUGIMURA, 1971). It is now well established that the polycyclic hydrocarbons are activated by microsomal hydroxylases in the liver and other tissues (NEBERT and GELBOIN, 1969) but less is known concerning the nature of the active intermediates although there is evidence that epoxide formation at the K region of molecules may occur (GROVER, SIMS, HUBERMAN, MARQUARDT, KUROKI and HEIDELBERGER, 1971). There is also evidence for microsomal metabolism of aflatoxins (SCHABORT and STEYN, 1969) and for binding of metabolites to cellular macromolecules (LIJINSKY, LEE and GALLAGHER, 1970) but detailed information on the chemistry of these reactions is lacking.

The N-dialkylnitrosamines undergo oxidative dealkylation *in vivo* to form alkylating agents which react with cellular macromolecules (MAGEE and HULTIN, 1962; MAGEE and FARBER, 1962) and the N-alkylnitrosamides appear to react in a similar manner without enzymic activation (SWANN and MAGEE, 1968, 1971) although there is evidence that in some cases the reaction is catalysed by sulphydryl compounds (SCHOENTAL and RIVE, 1965; LAWLEY and THATCHER, 1970). The original suggestion that the alkylating species were diazoalkanes is probably not correct in view of the findings of Lijinsky and his colleagues on the metabolism of fully deuterium-labelled dimethyl- and diethylnitrosamines. These authors observed that alkylated cellular components, in this case the 7-alkylguanines, isolated from livers of rats receiving the deuterated carcinogens had molecular weights corresponding to transference of the intact $-CD_3$ and $-CD_2CD_3$ groups respectively rather than $-CD_2H$ and $-CDHCD_3$ which would be formed if the diazoalkanes were obligatory intermediates (Lijinsky, Loo and Ross, 1968; Ross, Keefer and Lijinsky, 1971). This evidence favours the intermediate formation of the alkyl diazonium cations $CH_3CH_2N_2^+$ and $CH_3N_2^+$ and/or the corresponding carbonium ions $CH_3CH_2^+$ and CH_3^+ respectively. A similar reaction mechanism for N-methyl-N'-nitro-N-nitrosoguanidine is suggested by the work of Lingens, Haerlin and Sussmuth (1971) with the deuterated compound. There is evidence suggesting a similar final metabolic pathway for the naturally occurring carcinogen cycasin, $CH_3-\underset{\substack{\downarrow\\ O}}{N}=N-CH_2O$-glucose. This compound is activated by the microbial flora of the gastrointestinal tract, giving rise to methylazoxymethanol (MAM), $CH_3-\underset{\substack{\downarrow\\ O}}{N}=N-CH_2OH$ which is an alkylating agent *in vitro* (Matsumoto and Higa, 1966) and *in vivo* (Shank and Magee, 1967; Nagata and Matsumoto, 1969).

Several dialkylhydrazines, alkylazo and alkylazoxy compounds have been shown to be potent carcinogens by Druckrey and his colleagues (Druckrey, 1970) who suggested that this group of chemically related compounds might behave in a similar manner *in vivo* to cycasin and MAM and give rise to the same ultimate carcinogenic molecules (Druckrey, Preussmann, Ivankovic, Schmidt, So and Thomas, 1965). Considerable recent interest has been shown in 1,2-dimethylhydrazine which induces tumours of the colon in the rat (Druckrey, Preussmann, Matskies and Ivankovic, 1967), the mouse (Wiebecke, Lohrs, Gimmy and Eder, 1968) and the hamster (Osswald and Kruger, 1969). The metabolism of 1,2-dimethylhydrazine, 1,1-dimethylhydrazine and monomethylhydrazine has been studied *in vivo* and *in vitro* by Reed and his colleagues (Dost, Reed and Wang, 1966; Prough, Wittkop and Reed, 1969, 1970; Wittkop, Prough and Reed, 1969) who have reported that these compounds undergo oxidative dealkylation by liver microsomal preparations *in vitro*. Recent work in the laboratory of the author by Dr. A. Hawks and Dr. P. F. Swann has shown that 1,2-dimethylhydrazine alkylates DNA and RNA of mouse liver and colon *in vivo* (Hawks, Swann and Magee, 1972), thus providing experimental evidence that this group of carcinogens does react with cellular macromolecules in a manner similar to that of the nitroso compounds and the derivatives of methylazoxymethanol. The induction of tumours of the colon by 1,2-dimethylhydrazine in the mouse has been confirmed and squamous carcinomas of the anus were also found. In addition, administration of monomethylhydrazine to mice by repeated subcutaneous injection has been in progress for about 32 weeks, but no colonic or other tumour has so far been observed. In similar experiments with the 1,2-dimethyl compound tumours of the colon were already present in several mice after this period of administration so it appears that monomethylhydrazine may be considerably less potent as a colon carcinogen than the symmetrical dimethyl compound if, indeed, it induces colonic tumours at all. Treatment of mice with [^{14}C]monomethylhydrazine gave rise to some detectable methylation of nucleic acids but the extents of alkylation were very much lower than those with 1,2-dimethylhydrazine. It is of interest that unsymmetrical 1,1-dimethylhydrazine, which is only weakly carcinogenic, if at all (DRUCKREY *et al.*, 1961; ARGUS and HOCH-LIGETI, 1961; ROE, GRANT and MILLICAN, 1967) failed to produce detectable methylation of nucleic acids in rats to which it had been administered (KRUGER, WIESSLER and RUCKER, 1970). Taken together, these findings are consistent with the requirement for carcinogenesis of metabolic conversion of the precarcinogen to an electrophilic reactant.

Intracellular Targets for Ultimate Carcinogens

Apart from the work of FARBER and his colleagues on the binding of metabolites of 2-acetylaminofluorene to liver glycogen *in vivo* (EPSTEIN, MCNARY, BARTUS and FARBER, 1968) attention has been focussed on nucleic acids and proteins by most investigators because these macromolecules have been thought to be the only ones with sufficient molecular specificity to mediate the malignant transformation.

DNA

Since the malignant transformation requires a heritable change in the properties of the affected cells it has been thought by some authors that this could be mediated by a direct action of the ultimate carcinogen on the DNA of the cell to be transformed. Such a mechanism is, of course, consistent with well known somatic mutation hypothesis, first proposed by Boveri in 1895 (see papers by MARQUARDT, 1965; ZIMMERMANN, 1971; CORBETT, HEIDELBERGER and DOVE, 1970, for discussion). In the absence of means of formal genetic analysis of tumour cells, the hypothesis is virtually impossible to prove or disprove. Earlier objections (e.g., BURDETTE, 1955) that there was poor correlation between those chemicals which were carcinogenic and those which were mutagenic now have considerably less force with the recognition of the need for metabolic activation of precarcinogens. It is now known that many proximate and suggested ultimate carcinogens are, in fact, mutagenic (see MILLER and MILLER, 1971). Recent work from the laboratory of CHARLES HEIDELBERGER (CORBETT, HEIDELBERGER and DOVE, 1970) illustrates this approach to the validation of the somatic mutation hypothesis. These workers tested a number of carcinogens and some non-carcinogens for mutagenic activity in bacteriophage T4. The more chemically reactive compounds were found to be mutagenic in this system but there was no quantitative correlation between the effectiveness of the compound as a mutagen and its effectiveness as a carcinogen. The authors emphasise the desirability of testing for mutagenicity and carcinogenicity in the same *in vitro* system but point out that even completely consistent correlation would not constitute a final proof of whether the mechanism of chemical carcinogenesis involves a somatic mutation.

The results of some experiments by the writer and his colleagues with the carcinogen N-nitrosomethylurea may have a bearing on possible similarities between the mechanism of carcinogenesis and mutagenesis. This compound is powerfully mutagenic in a range of test organisms (see MAGEE and BARNES, 1967) and has recently been shown to induce reversions in four mutant auxotrophic strains of *E. Coli* by

Dr. STELLA NEALE, working in the laboratory of the author (NEALE, 1972). The compound is also a highly potent and versatile chemical carcinogen (DRUCKREY *et al.*, 1967) which will, under appropriate experimental conditions, induce tumours in most organs of the body, including the brain. Following single intragastric administration to rats tumours were induced in the stomach, small and large intestine, kidney, skin and in dental tissues (odontomas) (LEAVER, SWANN and MAGEE, 1969). Although the compound persists in the body for less than an hour, the half-life *in vivo* being only a few minutes (SWANN, 1968), it has time to become widely distributed throughout the body of the animal after administration as shown by whole-body autoradiography (KLEIHUES and PATZSCHKE, 1971). Also methylated nucleic acids, alkylated to about the same extent, were present in the different organs examined which included liver, kidney, lung, small and large intestine and spleen (SWANN and MAGEE, 1968). In most of the animals in the carcinogenesis study only one tumour was found and the greatest number observed in one rat was three. If it is assumed that each of these tumours could have been derived from a single aberrant cell, as is suggested by the work of FIALKOW, GARTLER and their colleagues (FIALKOW *et al.*, 1967, 1970) on chronic myeloid leukaemia and on Burkitt's lymphoma, it appears that malignant transformation *in vivo* by chemicals could be a very rare event indeed since the number of cells at risk in the animal body is enormous. It is, of course, probable that a number of abortive tumour cell clones may be formed only to be destroyed by the immunological defence mechanisms of the body, the process described by BURNET as immunosurveillance (see BURNET, 1969). That this is, in fact, the case is indicated by the detailed studies of HARD and BUTLER (1970, 1971) on the early stages of the dimethylnitrosamine induced rat kidney tumour.

Until recently the failure to detect ethylation of rat liver DNA by ethionine *in vivo* (FARBER, MCCONOMY and FRUMANSKI, 1967; ORTWERTH and NOVELLI, 1969) was considered by some to favour tRNA as a crucial intracellular target for chemical carcinogenesis (see below). Now, however, evidence has been obtained in the laboratory of the author that DNA, under certain experimental conditions, does appear to be ethylated by this carcinogen in rat liver *in vivo* since radioactive 7-ethylguanine was detected after administration of a relatively large single dose of [^{3}H]ethionine. Although the extent of this ethylation of DNA was very small (2.5pmol 7-ethylguanine/mg DNA or 1/230,000 guanine residues), a number of control experiments, notably the failure of equivalent doses of labelled methionine to produce any detectable 7-methylguanine in the liver DNA, supported the validity of the observation with ethionine (SWANN, PEGG, HAWKS, FARBER and MAGEE, 1971). The presence of 7-ethylguanine in the DNA of the target organ of ethionine treated animals does not, of course, imply any necessary correlation with carcinogenesis but it may be considered in the light of the comments of HEIDELBERGER *et al.* on the possible dose-related specificity of chemical carcinogens (CORBETT *et al.*, 1970). As pointed out by these authors, 0.004 pmole of 9,10-dimethyl-1,2-benzanthracene is equivalent in tumour-initiating potency to 240 μmoles of β-propiolactone in mouse skin, although 0.1 μmole of the hydrocarbon is bound per mole of DNA as compared with 400 μmoles of the lactone, i. e., there is a 4000-fold difference between the amounts of these compounds bound to DNA for an equivalent carcinogenic response. In a similar way there is a great difference in the extent of ethylation of rat liver DNA by ethionine and that by diethylnitrosamine (SWANN and MAGEE, 1971) and these results could be taken to indicate that interaction with DNA has no relation to carcinogenesis. Alternatively, however, they might suggest that there may be certain highly specific sites on the DNA molecule which are related to carcinogenesis and which are more readily accessible to reaction by some carcinogens than by others.

RNA and Protein

The possible importance of tRNA methylases in carcinogenesis was suggested by SRINIVASAN and BOREK (1963, 1964) and it was further suggested that tRNA might be a crucial target for chemical carcinogens (BOREK, 1963) because in some cases, notably that of ethionine, the carcinogen reacted more extensively with this than with other molecular species of RNA (FARBER, MCCONOMY, FRANZEN, MARROQUIN, STEWART and MAGEE, 1967; FARBER, MCCONOMY and FRUMANSKI, 1967; ORTWERTH and NOVELLI, 1969). The possible role of tRNA methylases in carcinogenesis has been recently discussed (CRADDOCK, 1970; MAGEE, 1971).

WEINSTEIN and his colleagues (WEINSTEIN, GRUNBERGER, FUJIMURA and FINK, 1971) have stressed the possible importance of tRNA as a target for chemical carcinogens. These authors point out that tumours may result from aberrations in differentiation which do not involve permanent changes in cellular DNA as implied in the somatic mutation hypothesis. In support of this concept WEINSTEIN points to the high efficiency of conversion of normal cells to tumour cells during *in vitro* chemical carcinogenesis which is difficult to reconcile with mutagenesis, the increasing number of proven cases of reversion to normal from the malignant state and expression in tumours of genes repressed during embryonic development. In detailed studies of the interaction of aromatic amine and azo dye carcinogens with tRNA a relative susceptibility of specific guanosine residues to modification by acetylaminofluorene was found. Conformational changes in the tRNA molecule were observed which the authors suggest might represent a general pattern for interaction of aromatic amine and polycyclic hydrocarbon carcinogens with nucleic acids. The reaction of the carcinogen N-nitrosomethylurea with tRNA *in vitro* has recently been investigated by Dr. A. E. PEGG in the laboratory of the author. In contrast to the observations of WEINSTEIN *et al.* mentioned above, PEGG could find no evidence for any specifically susceptible sites of methylation in the treated tRNA. Because of their relatively small molecular size tRNAs have obvious advantages as models for investigation of the interaction of carcinogens with nucleic acids but there does not appear to be any conclusive evidence to implicate them as crucial cellular targets in carcinogenesis.

The possible role of proteins as points of attack by chemical carcinogens is also unclear. As mentioned above, the first observation of an interaction between a carcinogen and a cellular constituent of a target organ was that between a metabolite of *p*-dimethylaminoazobenzene and rat liver protein *in vivo* (MILLER, E. C. and MILLER, J. A., 1947). In spite of very intensive subsequent study with azo dye and other chemical carcinogens (see MILLER, E. C. and MILLER, J. A., 1966; MILLER, J. A., 1970) the biological role of these interactions with proteins is still obscure. A very interesting recent development, however, has been the discovery of the protein ligandin (LITWACK, KETTERER and ARIAS, 1971). This protein, which occurs mainly in the liver, binds covalently and/or non-covalently with carcinogens, steroids, bilirubin and various exogenous organic anions. Carcinogens including azo dyes and methylcholanthrene differ from other compounds in that they bind covalently as well as non-covalently. Acetylaminofluorene, however, is not bound. What part ligandin may play in chemical carcinogenesis is not known but it has been suggested that this protein may have an important transport function determining the selective hepatic uptake of certain small molecules and perhaps influencing the flux of metabolites from the liver into the plasma or bile.

Conclusion

It is now firmly established that most, perhaps all, chemical carcinogens are electrophilic reactants or become converted into such reactants in the body. These so-called ultimate carcinogens react with nucleophilic centres in nucleic acids, proteins and probably other cellular components. An increasing number of them have been shown to be mutagenic. In view of the complexity of the various intracellular targets for carcinogens it is difficult to see how further detailed study of carcinogen-macromolecule interaction can lead to precise conclusions on the molecular mechanism of malignant transformation by chemicals. Recent advances in understanding of viral carcinogenesis (e. g., TEMIN, 1971) and the renewed interest in possible activation of latent oncogenic viruses or oncogenes (HUEBNER and TODARO, 1969) suggest that the way ahead for chemical carcinogenesis may be in the direction of investigation of its possible inter-relationship with viral carcinogenesis at the molecular level.

Acknowledgements

The author acknowledges the generous financial support of the Cancer Research Campaign of Great Britain.

References

ARGUS, M., HOCH-LIGETI, C.: J. nat. Cancer Inst. **27**, 695 (1961).
BOREK, E.: Quant. Biol. **28**, 139 (1963).
BURDETTE, W. J.: Cancer Res. **15**, 201 (1955).
BURNET, F. M.: Self and not-self. Melbourne and Cambridge: University Press 1969, p. 286.
CRADDOCK, V. M.: Nature (Lond.) **228**, 1264—1268 (1970).
CORBETT, T. H., HEIDELBERGER, C., DOVE, W. F.: Mol. Pharmacol. **6**, 667 (1970).
DOST, F. W., REED, D. J., WANG, C. H.: Biochem. Pharmacol. **15**, 1325 (1966).
DRUCKREY, H.: In: Carcinoma of the colon and antecedent epithelium. Ed.: W. J. BURDETTE. Illinois: Charles C. Thomas 1970, p. 267.
DRUCKREY, H., PREUSSMANN, R., IVANKOVIC, S., SCHMÄHL, D.: Z. Krebsforsch. **69**, 103 (1967).
DRUCKREY, H., PREUSSMANN, R., IVANKOVIC, S., SCHMIDT, C. H., SO, B. T., THOMAS, C.: Z. Krebsforsch. **67**, 31 (1965).
DRUCKREY, H., PREUSSMANN, R., MATZKIES, F., IVANKOVIC, S.: Naturwissenschaften **54**, 285 (1967).
DRUCKREY, H., PREUSSMANN, R., SCHMÄHL, D., MÜLLER, M.: Naturwissenschaften. **48**, 134 (1961).
EPSTEIN, S. M., MCNARY, J., BARTUS, B., FARBER, E.: Science **62**, 907 (1968).
FARBER, E., MCCONOMY, J., FRANZEN, B., MARROQUIN, F., STEWART, G. A., MAGEE, P. N.: Cancer Res. **27**, 1761 (1967).

FARBER, E., MCCONOMY, J., FRUMANSKI, B.: Proc. Amer. Ass. Cancer Res. **8**, 16 (1967).
FIALKOW, P. J., GARTLER S. M., YOSHIDA, A.: Proc. nat. Acad. Sci (Wash.) **58**, 1468 (1967).
FIALKOW, P. J., KLEIN, G., GARTLER, S. M., CLIFFORD, P.: Lancet **1970 I** 384.
GROVER, P. L., SIMS, P., HUBERMAN, H., MARQUARDT, H., KUROKI, T., HEIDELBERGER, C.: Proc. nat. Acad. Sci. (Wash.) **68**, 1098 (1971).
HARD, G. C., BUTLER, W. H.: Cancer Res. **30**, 2806 (1970).
HARD, G. C., BUTLER, W. H.: Cancer Res. **31**, 337 (1971).
HAWKS, A., SWANN, P. F., MAGEE, P. N.: Biochem. Pharmacol. **21**, 432 (1972).
HUEBNER, R., TODARO, G. J.: Proc. nat. Acad. Sci (Wash.) **64**, 1087 (1969).
KLEIHUES, P., PATZSCHKE, K.: Z. Krebsforsch. **75**, 193 (1971).
KRÜGER, F. W., WIESSLER, M., RÜCKER, U.: Biochem. Pharmacol. **19**, 1825 (1970).
LAWLEY, P. D., THATCHER, C. J.: Biochem. J. **116**, 693 (1970).
LEAVER, D. D., SWANN, P. F., MAGEE, P. N.: Brit. J. Cancer **23**, 177 (1969).
LIJINSKY, W., LEE, K. Y., GALLAGHER, C. H.: Cancer Res. **30**, 2280 (1970).
LIJINSKY, W., LOO, J., ROSS, A. E.: Nature (Lond.) **218**, 1174 (1968).
LINGENS, F., HAERLIN, R., SÜSSMUTH, R.: FEBS Letters **13**, 241 (1971).
LITWACK, G., KETTERER, B., ARIAS, I. M.: Nature (Lond.) **234**, 466 (1971).
MAGEE, P. N.: Cancer Res. **31**, 599 (1971).
MAGEE, P. N., BARNES, J. M.: Advanc. Cancer Res. **10**, 163 (1967).
MAGEE, P. N., FARBER, E.: Biochem. J. **83**, 114 (1962).
MAGEE, P. N., HULTIN, T.: Biochem. J. **83**, 106 (1962).
MARQUARDT, H.: Dtsch. med. Wschr. **90**, 398 (1965).
MATSUMOTO, H., HIGA, H. H.: Biochem. J. **98**, 20 c (1966).
MATSUSHIMA, T., SUGIMURA, T.: In: Chemistry and biological actions of 4-nitroquinoline 1-oxide. Eds.: H. ENDO. T. ONO, T. SUGIMURA. Berlin, Heidelberg and New York: Springer 1971, p. 53.
MILLER, E. C., MILLER, J. A.: Cancer Res. **7**, 468 (1947).
MILLER, E. C., MILLER, J. A.: Pharmacol. Rev. **18**, 805 (1966).
MILLER, E. C., MILLER, J. A.: In: Chemical Mutagens; principles and methods for their detection. Ed. A. HOLLAENDER. New York and London: Plenum Press 1971, Vol. 1, p. 83.
MILLER, J. A.: Cancer Res. **30**, 559 (1970).
MILLER, J. A., MILLER, E. C.: Lab. Invest. **15**, 217 (1966).
NAGATA, Y., MATSUMOTO, H.: Proc. Soc. exp. Biol. (N. Y.) **132**, 383 (1969).
NEALE, S.: Mutation Res. **14**, 155 (1972).
NEBERT, D. W., GELBOIN, H. V.: Arch. Biochem. Biophys. **134**, 76 (1969).
ORTWERTH, B. J., NOVELLI, G. D.: Cancer Res. **29**, 380 (1969).
OSSWALD, H., KRUGER, F. W.: Arzneimittel-Forsch. **19**, 1891 (1969).
PROUGH, R. A., WITTKOP, J. A., REED, D. J.: Biochim. biophys. Acta (Amst.) **131**, 369 (1969).
PROUGH, R. A., WITTKOP, J. A., REED, D. J.: Arch. Biochem. Biophys. **140**, 450 (1970).
ROE, F. J. C., GRANT, G. A., MILLICAN, D. M.: Nature (Lond.) **216**, 375 (1967).
ROSS, A. E., KEEFER, L., LIJINSKY, W.: J. nat. Cancer Inst. **47**, 789 (1971).
SCHABORT, J. C., STEYN, M.: Biochem. Pharmacol. **18**, 2241 (1969).
SCHOENTAL, R., RIVE, D. J.: Biochem. J. **97**, 466 (1965).
SHANK, R. C., MAGEE, P. N.: Biochem. J. **105**, 521 (1967).
SRINIVASAN, P. R., BOREK, E.: Proc. nat. Acad. Sci. (Wash.) **49**, 529 (1963).
SRINIVASAN, P. R., BOREK, E.: Science **145**, 548 (1964).
SWANN, P. F.: Biochem. J. **110**, 49 (1968).
SWANN, P. F., MAGEE, P. N.: Biochem. J. **110**, 39 (1968).
SWANN, P. F., MAGEE, P. N.: Biochem. J. **125**, 841 (1971).
SWANN, P. F., PEGG, A. E., HAWKS, A., FARBER, E., MAGEE, P. N.: Biochem. J. **123**, 175 (1971).
TEMIN, H. M.: J. nat. Cancer Inst. **46**, III (1971).
WIEBECKE, B., LÖHRS, U., GIMMY, J., EDER, M.: Z. ges. exp. Med. **149**, 277 (1969).
WITTKOP, J. A., PROUGH, R. A., REED, D. J.: Arch. Biochem. Biophys. **134**, 308 (1969).
ZIMMERMANN, F. K.: Biochem. Pharmacol. 20, 985 (1971).

Formation of Carcinogens From Precursors Occurring in the Environment: New Aspects of Nitrosamine - induced Tumorgenesis

R. PREUSSMANN

1. Introduction

Chemical carcinogens occurring in the environment are a major cause for human cancer. They include both substances arising from technical processes (e. g. polycyclic aromatic hydrocarbons such as 3,4-benzypyrene, released during combustion) and such "naturally occurring" substances as aflatoxin, a metabolite of a mold fungus, and various carcinogens of plant origin.

Systematic basic research has led to significant progress in the field of chemical carcinogens over the last 15—20 years, and the list of substances potentially dangerous to man has been considerably extended. The *organic N-nitro compounds* are typical examples; in 1956, MAGEE and BARNES [1] described the carcinogenic effect of dimethylnitrosamine in rats. Our group conducted large-scale structure-effect studies and was able to show that very many N-nitroso compounds exhibit pronounced carcinogenic effects [2]. The stage of pure basic research was quickly left behind when it became apparent that such compounds occur naturally; they were detected in microorganisms [3], lower [4] and higher [5] plants. Recently, simple nitrosamines have even been found in foodstuffs [6].

We had already indicated another way in which N-nitroso compounds might impair human health [7]; the example of tobacco smoke was used as an illustration of the possibility that nitrosamines might be formed from precursors. These precursors are secondary and tertiary amines and alkyl- or arylamides, and nitrosating agents such as nitrite, nitrous gases (NO and NO_2) or nitrate under reducing conditions. Such substances occur widely in the environment. ENDER *et al.* [8, 9] demonstrated the formation of dimethylnitrosamine in fishmeal treated with nitrite; J. SANDER, Tübingen, has made a particularly valuable contribution to progress in this field. The most important results will be summarized below.

2. Carcinogenic Effect of N-nitroso Compounds

Review articles on the carcinogenic effect of N-nitroso compounds have appeared [2, 10]. They are also known to have mutagenic, teratogenic and general toxic effects [10, 11]. Although direct demonstration of carcinogenesis in man has not yet been possible, it has been demonstrated in many different animal species, facilitating extrapolation to man: Dimethylnitrosamine was recognized as carcinogenic in 6 species, diethylnitrosamine in 12 species including subhuman primates [12, 13]. No animal species has yet been observed to possess any resistance to the carcinogenic effect of these or similar substances. Observations that dimethylnitrosamine and diethylnitrosamine can produce tumors in rodents when given in doses of about 1 mg/kg/day and below [14, 15] show the high level of biological efficiency. Very many nitrosamines and nitrosamides are carcinogenic after a *single* dose [2].

One outstanding characteristic of N-nitroso compounds is their capacity for inducing tumors in practically any important organ in mammals, the one selected being dependent on the chemical structure, and to some extent on the dosage, mode of administration and species. Liver, lung. stomach, esophagus, brain and nervous system, kidney and bladder are easily accessible to selective tumorgenesis [2, 10]. It must, therefore, be acknowledged that nitrosamines and nitrosamides are among the most potent and most versatile of all known chemical carcinogens.

3. Chemistry of the Nitrosation Reaction

General formula 1 shows the course of the nitrosation reaction of secondary amines and amides:

$$\begin{matrix} R_1 \\ R_2 \end{matrix}\!\!>N{\diagdown}H + HNO_2 \rightarrow \begin{matrix} R_1 \\ R_2 \end{matrix}\!\!>N-N=O + H_2O. \qquad \text{Form. 1}$$

The real nitrosating agent in this reaction is the NO^+ cation (formula 2), which is also active in nitrosation reactions with nitrous gases (formula 3).

$$2\,NO_2^- + 2\,H^+ \rightleftharpoons 2\,HNO_2 \rightleftharpoons O=N-O-N\!\begin{matrix} \nearrow O \\ \searrow O \end{matrix} + H_2O \rightleftharpoons NO^+ + NO_3^- \qquad \text{Form. 2}$$

$$NO + NO_2 \rightleftharpoons O=N-O-N\!\begin{matrix} \nearrow O \\ \searrow O \end{matrix} \rightleftharpoons NO^+ + NO_3^-. \qquad \text{Form. 3}$$

Nitrosation is thus effected by the NO^+ cation during reaction with the free electron pair of the amino compound. In the usual nitrosation reactions with nitrites an acid pH is necessary according to formula 2. As, however, in the basic amines the free electron pair is largely occupied with protonation at acid pH and is thus not susceptible to nitrosation with NO^+, the following conclusions are possible:

a) the nitrosation of secondary amines in aqueous solutions is pH-dependent;

b) the more basic an amine is, the more difficult is nitrosation at acid pH; the more weakly basic any amine or amide is, the more easily it will react with nitrous acid.

The optimum pH for nitrosation of diethylamine with nitrite is 3.4, which is close to the disassociation constant of 3.37 for nitrous acid [16].

Mirvish [17] examined nitrosation kinetics in 4 secondary amines at pH 3.0. At this level the relative speed of nitrosation is expressed by the reaction constant k_2, which is clearly dependent on the basicity of the amine, expressed as the pK_a of the amine (Table 1).

The nitrosation of piperazine, as the amine with the lowest basicity, thus takes place 185,000 times faster than that of the very basic amine piperazine. Sander *et al.* [18] obtained similar results. The main difference in the reactions between

Table 1. Reaction constants k_2 of the nitrosation of secondary amines with different basicity (adapted from MIRVISH)

Amine	pK_a	K_2
Piperidine	11.2	0.027
Dimethylamine	10.7	0.1
Morpholine	8.7	14.8
Mononitrosopiperazine	6.8	400
Piperazine	5.57	5000

nitrous acid and various amines thus lies in the proportion of amine not protonated at a given pH, which in turn is dependent on the basicity of the amine concerned. Alkylamides are very rapidly nitrosated (SANDER [18]); the reaction has been examined in detail by MIRVISH [19]. As amides possess practically no basicity there is no optimum pH value for the reaction. The reaction constants therefore only vary by a factor of about 25 between methyl urea and hydantoin.

Contrary to popular opinion even among chemists, tertiary amines can also be converted to nitrosamines if one alkyl group is split off. LIJINSKY [20] recently examined this reaction in detail using various major drugs, and indicated the possible dangers of this sort of reaction in the human stomach.

Model Experiments *in vitro* and *in vivo*

The above discussion shows that the formation of N-nitroso compounds is most likely to occur in the mammalian stomach where the pH is predominantly acid. There is now a considerable amount of evidence that N-nitroso compounds can be formed in these conditions. SANDER *et al.* [21, 22] have shown that various secondary amines are nitrosated by nitrite in gastric juice. SEN *et al.* [23] obtained similar results: they used diethylamine + nitrite to show that the gastric juice of man and rabbit, with a pH of 1—2, forms more nitrosamine than that of rat, which has a pH of 4—5. A pH which is not favourable to nitrosation can, however, be compensated by a rise in the nitrite concentration. Thus ASAHINA *et al.* [24] were able to show that dimethylnitrosamine was formed in the stomach of mouse following high doses of nitrite, as was apparent from typical acute toxic effects of nitrosamines. The formation of methylnitrosourea from the amide and nitrite was recognized by the characteristic methylation of nucleic acid in stomach, liver and small intestine of rats [25].

The stomach, with its acid pH, is not, however, the only site of carcinogen formation: both SANDER [26] and HAWKSWORTH and HILL [27] have shown in *in vitro* tests that bacteria present in the normal intestinal flora can act as catalysts in the nitrosation of secondary amines *at neutral pH values*. These are enterobacteria and other species which reduce nitrates, and they cannot use only nitrite in the nitrosation reaction, but also *nitrate*. Accordingly, ALAM *et al.* [28] were able to demonstrate the formation of N-nitrosopiperidine from nitrate and piperidine in the gastrointestinal tract of rats *in vivo*. It is known that dimethylnitrosamine is also formed in similar circumstances [29].

Table 2. Tumor production in experimental animals by simultaneous oral administration of secondary amino compounds and nitrite (numbers in brackets refer to references)

Animal species	Amino compound	Nitrosating agent	Tumors in	Expected tumor localization
Rat	methylaniline	$NaNO_2$	oesophagus [30]	oesophagus [2]
Rat	morpholine	$NaNO_2$	liver [30]	liver [2]
Rat	methylbenzylamine	$NaNO_2$	oesophagus [30]	oesophagus [2]
Mouse	methylbenzylamine	$NaNO_2$	forestomach, oesophagus [30]	?
Mouse	morpholine	$NaNO_2$	lung (adenomas) [30]	lung (adenomas) [31]
Mouse	piperazine	$NaNO_2$	lung (adenomas) [31]	lung (adenomas) [31]
Mouse	methylaniline	$NaNO_2$	lung (adenomas) [31]	lung (adenomas) [31]
Rat	methylurea	$NaNO_2$	brain (nervous system) [32]	brain (nervous system) [2]
Rat	N,N'-dimethylurea	$NaNO_2$	brain (nervous system) [32]	brain (nervous system) [2]
Rat	imidazolidinone	$NaNO_2$	kidney, parotis [32]	?
Rat (transplacental)	ethylurea	$NaNO_2$	brain, nervous system [33]	brain, nervous system [2, 34]

Carcinogenicity Tests

Numerous results have now been published showing that simultaneous oral administration of secondary amines or amides and nitrite to experimental animals leads to tumors typical of the N-nitroso compounds concerned. Neither nitrite alone nor amino compounds alone have yet led to formation of tumors in corresponding control experiments.

Table 2 shows some important results. The list is not complete and only typical examples are selected.

The results given herewith show unequivocally that, when tumors are induced by giving an amino compound capable of nitrosation and nitrite simultaneously in the diet, they occur at exactly the same sites as those induced with the corresponding N-nitroso compound. In the *in vitro* tests, the occurrence of the corresponding nitrosamines and nitrosamides was directly detected by analysis; taken together with these results, the animal experiments prove conclusively that carcinogenic N-nitroso compounds can be formed by corresponding substances which are not themselves carcinogenic.

An experimental procedure particularly suitable for the resolution of a number of problems is transplacental carcinogenesis; by treating pregnant animals with ethyl urea and nitrite during the second half of the pregnancy we [33] were able to induce tumors in the brain and nervous system of the offspring which were typical of those formed by the corresponding ethylnitrosourea. The results are seen in Table 3. No tumors were induced in control tests with nitrite only or ethyl urea only.

Table 3. Transplacental induction of malignant tumors in rats by treatment of mothers during second half of pregnancy with ethylurea and sodium nitrite [33]

Age of death (days)	Diagnosis
77	Myelo-monocytary leukemia
133	Malig. neurinoma of the left n. trigeminus and of the Cauda equina
167	Malig. neurinoma of the right n. trigeminus and Ganglion Gasseri
168	Mixed glioma of the brain (Oligo-astrocytoma)
169	Malig. neurinoma of the right n. trigeminus
175	Medulloblastoma in the brain
176	Malignant neurinomas in plexus brachialis, lumbosacralis and n. femoralis r.
196	Malignant neurinoma of plexus lumbosacralis r.
204	Malig. neurinoma of n. trigeminus r., plexus brachialis l. and n. ischiadicus r.
211	Malig. neurinoma of n. trigeminus r., n. vagus r. and cauda equina

Conclusions

The studies performed so far leave no room for doubt that carcinogenic N-nitroso compounds can arise from appropriate precursors in the gastrointestinal tract of man and other mammals. The acid milieu of the stomach provides particularly favourable conditions for this chemical reaction; in the presence of certain entero-bacteria nitrosamine synthesis can even take place at a neutral pH and when nitrate is used. Nitrites are present in man's environment and are allowed as food preservatives and food additives in many countries. Nitrates occur almost everywhere, and are particularly widespread in soil and water, and also in plants. They are widely used as nitrogenous fertilizers in agriculture. Amino compounds capable of nitrosation are also widely distributed and also occur in many foodstuffs. It is thus very probable that these substances constitute a health risk if they come together within the organism.

Investigations in this new field of cancer research are still in the early stages. Systematic investigations on the environmental occurrence of nitrites and nitrates and of amino compounds capable of nitrosation, particularly in foodstuffs, have yet to be performed. The time the precursors remain in the gastrointestinal tract also needs further study. Prophylactic measures are possible, for example, reduction or discontinuation of the use of nitrites as food additives.

Summary

The experimental evidence for the formation of carcinogenic N-nitroso compounds from appropriate precursors is reviewed and the consequences are discussed.

References

1. MAGEE, P. N., BARNES, J. M.: Brit. J. Cancer **10**, 114 (1956).
2. DRUCKREY, H., PREUSSMANN, R., IVANKOVIC, S., SCHMÄHL, D.: Z. Krebsforsch. **69**, 103 (1967).
3. HERR, R. R., JAHNKE, H. K., ARGOUDEUS, A. D.: J. Amer. chem. Soc. **89**, 4808 (1967).
4. HERMANN, H.: Z. physiol. Chem. **326**, 13 (1961).
5. DU PLESSIS, L. S., NUNN, J. R., ROACH, W. A.: Nature (Lond.) **222**, 1198 (1969).
6. FAZIO, T., WHITE, R. H., HOWARD, J. W.: J. Ass. off. anal. Chem. **54**, 1157 (1971).
7. DRUCKREY, H., PREUSSMANN, R.: Naturwissenschaften **49**, 498 (1962).
8. ENDER, F., HAVRE, G., HELGEBOSTAD, A., KOPPANG, N., MADSEN, R., CEH, L.: Naturwissenschaften **51**, 637 (1964).
9. SAKSHAUG, J., SÖGNEN, E., HANSEN, M. A., KOPPANG, N.: Nature (Lond.) **206**, 1261 (1965).
10. MAGEE, P. N., BARNES, J. M.: Advanc. Cancer Res. **16**, 163 (1967).
11. MAGEE, P. N.: Fd. Cosmet. Toxiol. **9**, 207 (1971).
12. IARC-Monographes of the Evaluation of Chemicals to Man. Vol. 1, Lyon 1972.
13. SCHMÄHL, D., OSSWALD, H.: Experientia (Basel) **23**, 497 (1968).
14. TERRACINI, B., MAGEE, P. N., BARNES, J. M.: Brit. J. Cancer **21**, 559 (1967).
15. DRUCKREY, H., SCHILDBACH, A., SCHMÄHL, D., PREUSSMANN, R., IVANKOVIC, S.: Arzneimittel-Forsch. **13**, 841 (1963).
16. MIRVISH, S. S.: J. nat. Cancer Inst. **44**, 633 (1970).
17. MIRVISH, S. S.: IARC Sci. Publ. No 3., Lyon 1972.
18. SANDER, J., BÜRKLE, G., FLOHE, L., AEIKENS, B.: Arzneimittel-Forsch. **21**, 411 (1971).
19. MIRVISH, S. S.: J. nat. Cancer Inst. **46**, 1183 (1971).
20. LIJINSKY, W.: IARC Sci. Publ. No 3., Lyon 1972.
21. SANDER, J.: Arch. Hyp. Bakt. **151**, (1967).
22. SANDER, J., SCHWEINSBERG, F., MENZ, H. P.: Z. physiol. Chem. **349**, 1691 (1968).
23. SEN, N. P., SMITH, D. C., SCHWINGHAMMER, L.: Fd. Cosmet. Toxiol. **7**, 301 (1969).
24. ASAHINA, S., FRIEDMAN, M. A., ARNOLD, E., MILLAR, G. N., MISHKIN, M., BISOP, Y., EPSTEIN, S. S.: Cancer Res. **31**, 1201 (1971).

25. MONTESANO, R., MAGEE, P. N.: Intern. J. Cancer **7**, 249 (1971).
26. SANDER, J.: Z. physiol. Chem. **349**, 429 (1968).
27. HAWKSWORTH, G. M., HILL, M. J.: Brit. J. Cancer **25**, 520 (1971).
28. ALAM, B. S., SAPOROSCHETZ, I. B., EPSTEIN, S. S.: Nature (Lond.) **232**, 199 (1971).
29. KLUBES, P., JONDORF, W. R.: Res. Comm. Chem. Pathol. Pharmacol. **2**, 24 (1971).
30. SANDER, J.: Arzneimittel-Forsch. **21**, 1572 (1971).
31. GREENBLATIN, M., MIRVISH, S. S., SO, B. T.: J. nat. Cancer Inst. **46**, 1029 (1971).
32. SANDER, J.: Arzneimittel-Forsch. **21**, 1707 (1971).
33. IVANKOVIC, S., PREUSSMANN, R.: Naturwissenschaften **57**, 460 (1970).
34. IVANKOVIC, S., DRUCKREY, H.: Z. Krebsforsch. **71**, 320 (1968).

Intrauterine Induction of Cancer by the Experimental Application of Chemical Substances

S. IVANKOVIC

In 1971 a number of papers were published by GREENWALD and HERBST [1, 2, 3], which may be regarded as the first evidence of an intrauterine, i. e. prenatal, carcinogenic effect of chemical substances in humans. In approximately 14 females between 15 and 22 years of age, the mothers of whom had been treated with synthetic estrogens (diethylstilboestrol) during the first trimenon of pregnancy, the authors observed adenocarcinomas of the vagina. This supports the assumption that malignant growths can also be induced transplacentally in humans by a single or repeated application of chemical substances.

In many animal experiments carried out in recent years it has been determined that malignant growths may be produced in various organs if the mother animals come into contact with certain chemicals during the gestational period. So far, some 25 chemical agents have become known to us, which may induce cancer transplacentally in the descendants of various animal species treated with these agents in experiments (Table).

LARSEN was the first to succeed in producing pulmonary adenomas in the descendants of female mice which had been treated with urethan during the gestational period [4]. His findings were later confirmed and supplemented by a number of other authors [5, 6, 7].

In 1961, GELSHTEIN was able to induce malignant hepatomas and pulmonary adenomas in mice by transplacental application of orthoaminoazotoluene [8]. In 1962, DRUCKREY and STEINHOFF observed a diffuse carcinomatosis of the liver in a young guinea pig, the mother of which had been treated with diethylnitrosamine during the entire period of gestation [9].

In 1965, MOHR *et al.* published their observations of the incidence of tracheapapillomas among the descendants of hamsters after the pregnant mother animals had been treated with diethylnitrosamine [10]. In the same year we succeeded in inducing malignant tumours of the nervous system of the rat by diaplacental transfer [11, 12, 13]. In these experiments, the pregnant mothers received one or several doses of ethyl-nitroso urea (ENU) during the second half of the gestational period. A few months after birth, almost all the descendants died of malignant growths in the brain, the spinal medullary or of the nerves.

Pathohistological examinations showed that mainly mixed gliomas (oligo-astrocytomas) were to be found in the brain and the spinal medullary. In approximately 15% of all cases, more or less differentiated ependymomas were observed. In the

Table. Chemical substances with a diaplacental carcinogenic effect in experiments and humans

ethyl-carbamat (urethane)
ethyl-nitroso-biuret
ethyl-nitroso-urea
azoethane
azoxyethane
3,4-benzpyrene
n-butyl-nitroso-urea
cycas-flour (methyl-azoxy-methanol)
1,2-diethyl-hydrazine
diethyl-sulfate
diethyl-nitrosamine
7,12-dimethyl-benz(a)anthrazene
dimethyl-nitrosamine
methylcholantrene
methyl-nitroso-urea
1-methyl-2-benzyl-hydrazine
Natulan, (N-isopropyl-α-2-(methyl-hydrazino)-p-toluamide)
1-phenyl-3,3-diethyl-triazene
1,3-propansultone
1-pyridyl-3,3 — diethyl-triazene
^{32}P
n-propyl-nitroso-urea
stilbestrol (in humans)

case of the nerves, we found malignant neurinomas of Antoni types A and B and so-called "neurosarcomas".

In this context, we consider it to be of particular significance that ependymomas occurred in the cerebrum of the descendants. When the same substance was applied to adult rats such ependymomas were observed only in a few cases. It is known from human pathology that ependymomas located in the cerebral hemispheres are the most common glioma during youth. This striking parallel might therefore imply that this type of growth is also induced prenatally in humans.

Extremely small doses of ENU proved to be sufficient for cancerising the descendants. Chart 1 illustrates the ratio of doses and their effectiveness, and the tumour yield of neurogenic malignant growths among the descendants of the individual dose groups (expressed in per cent) has been entered in a logarithmic table of probability. In this way, we arrived at a liner regression (A). The average carcinogenic dose of ENU as shown in the chart is 3.2 milligrams/kg, which is a very low figure indeed (approximately 1.3% of LD 50). Another interesting fact is that the effectiveness rating line drops quite slowly, which gives us reason to believe that there is still a considerably high degree of effectiveness even if the doses applied are even smaller. For the sake of comparison, we then examined the effect of ENU applied once on adult rats of the same strain (BD IX). The result of this examination, again expressed in terms of the percentage yield of neurogenic tumours, is shown by regression line B, which illustrates that the average effective dose of ENU inducing neurogenic malignant growths among half of the adult rats, is 160 milligrams/kg. Thus, it is approximately 50 times higher than the dose required during prenatal development. This result, using carcinogenic ENU as an example, shows in a very impressive manner how sensitively the nervous system reacts to certain carcinogenic noxes in prenatal stages.

During prenatal development, the degree of sensitivity of the neurogenic tissue varies. When examining the effect of a single dose of ENU applied on different days during gestation, we arrived at the surprising result that hardly any carcinogenic effect at all can be determined on the 12th day of prenatal development, whereas it is lacking completely on the 11th day or the days before that. The starting point

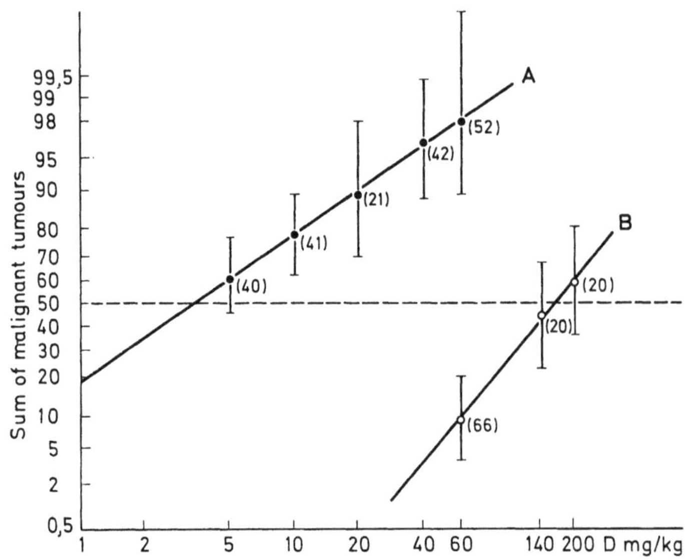

Fig. 1. Effectiveness ratings showing the induction of neurogenic malignant growths by a single dose of ethyl-nitroso urea
Line A: during fetal development (day 15 p. c.)
Line B: in adult rats

is particularly noticeable, because as from day 13 onwards ENU induced neurogenic malignant growths in practically all of the descendants, but did not do so in any of them before day 12. The examination carried out involved more than 1,500 rats, so that the result may be regarded as conclusive. The question why no malignant growths were induced during the first 12 days, whereas sensitivity suddenly increased on day 13, has not been answered so far. In fact, there are various ways of interpreting this striking difference, the first interpretation being that no effect is possible until the placenta has been connected. However, the placenta is already connected on the 11th day of gestation. Moreover, Spatz and Laqueur [14] have conducted experiments in which a few tumours were found in the brains of descendants, the mothers of which had been treated with cycasine on days 2—5 of gestation, i. e. long before placentation. This proves that, in principle, neurogenic tumours may certainly be induced during early embryonal development as well.

Thus, the second interpretation might be that at this early stage the nerve tissue is not yet sensitive enough. This conclusion might be drawn from the results SPATZ and LAQUEUR arrived at, since they found tumours of the brain only among a limited number of descendants. The third interpretation would be that the carcinogen is activated by catalytic or enzymatic processes which, in the course of embryonal or fetal development, only become possible after the 12th day.

It is this concept that leads us to the problem of the various enzymatic and catalytic potencies occurring in the course of ontogenetic development. By examining various carcinogenic substances, the activation mechanisms of which are known, we now have new possibilities of looking into this matter in a systematic way. In fact, we have already started carrying out such experiments and have arrived at some interesting results. The example we would like to quote here is that dialkylnitrosamines, which are very effective carcinogens in the case of adult animals, did not induce cancer in the descendants in one single case when applied to the mother on day 15 of prenatal development. The hydroxylases required for dealkylating or activating these substances are only produced shortly before birth or thereafter. A large oral dose of diethylnitrosamine applied to the mother animals shortly before birth induced cancer of the liver among approximately 60% of the descendants [15]. However, this cancer did not occur until the end of the descendants' life-span, i. e. after an average induction period of 850 days. This proves that a malignant growth occurring at old age might well have been caused originally during the prenatal stages of development. In addition, this example is also able to show that cancer can be induced transplacentally in other organs as well, and not only in the nervous system. It has in the meantime been possible to produce malignant growths diaplacentally in the kidney [16], the esophagus [17], the lung [18], and the thyroid gland [19] of animals, by applying various chemical carcinogens. It follows from this that the transplacental induction of cancer does not only depend on the degree of sensitivity and reactibility of the biological target, but also on the chemical structure of the carcinogen. The extent to which the chemical properties of the carcinogen influence its transplacental effectiveness is made clear by the fact that ethyl compounds are much more active than the corresponding methyl derivatives. This difference has been shown very clearly by our transplacental experiments with rats using 1,2-diethylhydrazine, azoethane, azoxyethane [20] and 1-phenyl- or 1-pyridyl-3,3-diethyl-triazene [21], as compared with experiments in which we used the corresponding methyl derivatives.

In conclusion, I would like to report on the transplacental carcinogenic effect of Natulan (registered trademark) (procarbazine). Natulan ® (N-isopropyl-α-2 (methylhydrazino)-p-toluamid) is used as a therapeutic agent for treating certain malignant growths. In experiments, Natulan has proved to be carcinogenic even when applied in single doses only. The fact that Natulan is used for a number of purposes also in the case of young people suffering from chronical hepatitis, lupus erythematodes visceralis, hemolytic anemia and Dupuytren's contracture, induced us to apply Natulan in a transplacental experiment in order to examine its carcinogenic effect. In so doing, we found that a single intravenous dose of Natulan, given to rats at the end of the gestational period, caused all the descendants to die of malignant neurogenic tumours at a young age, i. e. between the 5th and the 12th month after birth [22].

It follows from this fact that drugs with a potential carcinogenic effect should be applied only in the case of vital indications (SCHMÄHL [23]). This applies particularly to pregnant women and young people.

References

1. GREENWALD, P., BARLOW, J. J., NASCA, P. C., BURNETT, W. S.: New Engl. J. Med. **285,** 390 (1970).
2. HERBST, A. L., ULFELDER, H., POSKANZER, D. C.: New Engl. J. Med. **284,** 878 (1971).
3. HERBST, A. L., ULFELDER, H., POSKANZER, D. C.: New Engl. J. Med. **285,** 407 (1971).
4. LARSEN, C. D.: J. nat. Cancer Inst. **8,** 63 (1947).
5. KLEIN, M.: J. nat. Cancer Inst. **12,** 1003 (1952).
6. SMITH, W. E., ROUS, P.: J. exp. Med. **88,** 529 (1948).
7. VESSELINOVITCH, S. D., MIHAILOVITCH, N., PIETRA, G.: Cancer Res. **27,** 2333 (1967).
8. GELSHTEIN, V. I.: Vop. Onkol. **7,** 58 (1961).
9. DRUCKREY, H., STEINHOFF, D.: Naturwissenschaften **49,** 21, 497 (1962).
10. MOHR, U., ALTHOFF, J., WRBA, H.: Z. Krebsforsch. **66,** 526 (1965).
11. IVANKOVIC, S.: Deutscher Krebskongreß, München (1966).
12. IVANKOVIC, S., DRUCKREY, H.: Z. Krebsforsch., 320 (1968).
13. IVANKOVIC, S.: Habil. Schrift Freiburg/Br. 1968.
14. SPATZ, M., LAQUEUR, G. L.: J. nat. Cancer Inst. **38,** 233 (1967).
15. IVANKOVIC, S.: The Second Intern. Symp. of the Princess Takamatsu Cancer Research Fund Nov. Tokyo 1971.
16. ALEXANDROV, V. A.: Nature (Lond.) **218,** 280 (1968).
17. LIHACEV, A. Y.: Vop. Onkol. **17,** 45 (1971).
18. TOMATIS, L., TURUSOV, V., GUIBBERT, D., DUPERRAY, B., MALAVEILLE, C., PACHECO, H.: J. nat. Cancer Inst. **47,** 645 (1971).
19. NAPALKOV, N. P.: IARC Scientific Publication Vol. 4, p. 1, 1972.
20. DRUCKREY, H., IVANKOVIC, S., PREUSSMANN, R., LANDSCHÜTZ, C., STEKAR, J., BRUNNER, U., SCHAGEN, B.: Experientia (Basel) **24,** 561 (1968).
21. DRUCKREY, H.: In: Transplacental Carcinogenesis. IARC Scientific Publication, Vol. 4, p. 45, 1972.
22. IVANKOVIC, S.: IARC Scientific Publication, Vol. 4, p. 92, 1972.
23. SCHMÄHL, D., OSSWALD, H.: Arzneimittel-Forsch. **20,** 1461 (1970).

The Replication of RNA Tumor Viruses

K. von der Helm

The essential requirement for studying the molecular biology of cancer cells is a tool which can change normal cells into cancer cells. Fortunately, this tool is provided by nature itself; cancer is induced upon infection by certain viruses. There are DNA and RNA-containing viruses which can transform normal cells into malignant cells as Dr. Pontén pointed out.

DNA-viruses like polyoma, SV40 and adeno can induce cancer experimentally in animals and cell cultures; although it is not known whether they are natural causes of cancer. This report will deal with RNA tumor viruses. They include authentic models of natural leukemias and sarcomas in avian and vertebrate animals (perhaps also in man). Of these viruses, Rous virus causing sarcomas in chicken is the most studied one.

It is likely that the introduction of new genetic material (the viral nucleic acid) plays a key role in transforming a normal cell to a cancer cell. Therefore, the main question is the relationship of the viral genome to the cell genome in infected cells. Here, however, we remain in the dark.

The fate of the viral RNA during its replication within the host cell may involve a special biochemical pathway. Historically the "path-way" of its elucidation climaxed almost two years ago in the finding of an RNA dependent DNA polymerase in RNA tumor viruses. This permitted *in vitro* experiments necessary to test Temin's hitherto heretical hypothesis of the RNA replication pathway: RNA → DNA intermediate → RNA. In the first fever of excitement, those viruses infected and transformed no longer only animal cells but whole laboratories into proselytes of RNA tumor virology.

The golden age seemed to have arrived but after these past two years of paper production it now appears not to be that golden. Let us discuss some facts of the replication of RNA tumor viruses.

Some RNA viruses — the cytocidal viruses-infect cells force them to replicate the viral RNA via an *RNA-RNA* intermediate and then kill the host cell.

The Pro-Virus Hypothesis

However, the RNA tumor viruses do not fall into this category. They do not kill their hosts but transform them to cancer cells. Indirect evidence suggests that the mechanism of RNA tumor virus replication differs from that of cytocidal RNA virus in three distinct properties:

1. Permanent requirement for DNA dependent RNA synthesis [1, 2].
2. The possible early requirement for virus specific DNA synthesis [3, 4].
3. The requirement for cellular DNA synthesis and mitosis [5, 6, 7].

These peculiar properties led TEMIN to postulate a DNA intermediate in RNA tumor virus replication which he called the "pro virus", analogous to bacteriophage DNA integration as a prophage [1, 8]. This pro virus intermediate is postulated to be made by reverse transcription of viral RNA and to be integrated into the cellular chromosome. This may permanently transform a cell so that it practically never reverts to the normal state. The pro virus DNA can then replicate together with the host gene and is supposed to serve as a template for synthesis of progeny viral RNA.

TEMIN himself began the search for the virus specific DNA in infected cells. He compared viral RNA with the DNA of virus-transformed cells and DNA of uninfected cells using molecular hybridization [8]. However, there were two problems. One was a high background of nonspecific annealing. Secondly, the difference in annealing between viral RNA and DNA from normal and cancer cells turned out to be too small to confirm the pro virus hypothesis. These hybridization experiments were repeated many times by other tumor virologists — always with new courage. The results remained more or less the same, the interpretations, however, alternated [9, 13]. The majority finally concluded that a least some DNA complementary to viral RNA is integrated into the cellular genome of infected and — also of uninfected cells. We will discuss these amazing results later.

RNA Dependent DNA Polymerase

In the meantime a RNA → DNA synthesizing enzyme was found in the virus by TEMIN and BALTIMORE, working independently [14, 15]. This was immediately loved by virologists and many molecular biologists, because it offered a simple way to explain RNA tumor virus replication and supported the pro virus hypothesis.

If we review the experiments that were done in order to study RNA tumor virus replication *in vitro*, we end up with some results that support and other results that do not support the biological role of DNA polymerase in virus replication.

Properties of the Enzyme that Favor the Replicase Role

1. The ubiquity of the enzyme in all known infectious forms of RNA tumor viruses, while it is not found in other RNA viruses [16, 17, see ref. 18].
2. The ability of at least the unpurified enzyme to transcribe most of the viral RNA to DNA, measured by molecular hybridization of viral RNA and the *in vitro* DNA product [19].
3. The presence of at least one enzyme molecule per virion [20].
4. The preference of 60-70S tumor virus RNA as the best RNA-template for the enzyme among natural RNAs tested [20, 21].

Properties that do not Support the Replicase Role

1. The chain length of the DNA product is much smaller than the viral RNA template [16, 19, 22, 23].
2. The rate of DNA synthesis is very low (net synthesis) [20, 23].

3. The enzyme requires a primer; the DNA product is not initiated de novo, but covalently linked to the primer and not released from the template-primer [21, 23, 24, 35].

Nevertheless, this does not exclude the postulated role of the enzyme in virus replication, since all these experiments were done *in vitro*. Conditions *in vivo* may involve more complex reactions.

Since the introduction of the viral genome to a cell plays a key role in transforming a normal cell into a cancer cell, our discussion about the replication of tumor virus RNA will now focus on the nature of the viral RNA itself. This will aid us in understanding the above mentioned facts: 1. that 60-70S RNA is the best RNA template for this enzyme, 2. that a primer is required and 3. that there is covalent binding of the DNA product to the primer.

The RNA of RSV

Rous, like other RNA tumor viruses, has a high molecular-weight single-stranded RNA that sediments at 60-70S and a heterogeneous population of small size RNA's with a sedimentation constant of 4-8S [25].

The large RNA is thought to be the viral genome; the purpose of the small RNA is unknown; part of that RNA may be of cellular origin. Upon treatment with heat or DMSO the 60-70S RNA dissociates into smaller subunits (30-40S) [26, 27] and very small RNA (3-10S) that differs from the abovementioned small RNAs [28].

The subunits are thought to be linked together by hydrogen bonds to form the 60-70S RNA (Fig. 1). Along this large single stranded RNA the small RNA is bound to complementary regions; generating partly double stranded regions which might be sites for initiation of DNA synthesis. The 3' ends of these small RNAs might act as a primer for the viral DNA polymerase, which links the DNA covalently to these small RNAs [24].

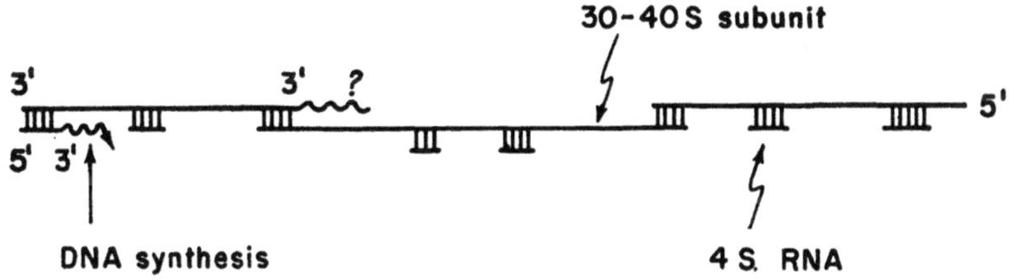

Fig. 1. Hypothetical model of 60-70S Rous sarcoma virus RNA used as template for DNA synthesis

HEATING melts the partly double stranded structure of the 60-70S RNA and reduces its template activity for the polymerase about 10-fold [20]. Thus heated Rous sarcoma virus (= RSV) RNA may be similar in its structure to other single stranded RNAs which also exhibit poor template activity for the RSV DNA polymerase.

M. LAI in our laboratory found that the Rous 60-70S RNA contains several polyadenylic acid rich regions of about 160 adenylic acid residues in length [29]. About

2.5% of the 60-70S RNA consists of Poly A. Functions of these Poly A regions are not yet clear. They may have a direct control function or they may be message which is to be transcribed.

Is Poly A a Preferred DNA Initiation Site

A possible role for the poly A regions is suggested by the following *in vitro* experiment. We have found that the template activity of 60-70S Rous RNA is enhanced 2—3 times upon addition of Oligo T and Oligo dC [21] (Table 1). It is known that Oligo T and to a lesser extent Oligo dC is bound to poly A [30]. A possible explanation is that these oligodeoxynucleotides bind to poly A regions within the 60-70S RNA and that these partially double stranded regions can function as primers for RSV DNA polymerase. In order to test this hypothesis we annealed poly U quantitatively to 60-70S RNA, thus covering all poly A regions (Table 2). As expected, no stimulation of template activity was observed (Table 2). Poly U or Oligo U does not function as a primer under the conditions we used [31]. Using RNA annealed to poly U as template (no Oligo T) we observed a 60% decrease in DNA synthesis compared to 100% activity using native 60-70S RNA as template.

Table 1. Stimulation of TMP incorporation by Oligo deoxynucleotides

Oligonucleotide		pmole TMP incorp./60 min
1 μg 60-70S RNA	no	5.2
1 μg 60-70S RNA	0.1 μg Oligo T	13.2
1 μg 60-70S RNA	0.1 μg Oligo dC	12.1

Preparation of the polymerase and standard DNA polymerase assay are described in references 20 and 21. A standard assay contained in 100 μl solution: 50 mM Tris (pH 8.0), 50 mM KCl, 5 mM dithiothreitol, 6 mM $MgCl_2$, three unlabeled dNTPs at 0.1 mM and one [^{3}H] dNTP at 2 μM (10—15 ci/mmole). 1 μg of RNA was used as template, and about 0.05 μg of enzyme protein. The incubation was terminated by addition of 2 ml 5% trichloracetic acid, the acid insoluble material collected on Millipore filters and these filters counted in a liquid scintillation counter.

Table 2. Poly U hybridization to 60-70S RNA

			Pmole TMP incorp/60 min	
	0.5 μg 60-70S RNA	Poly U	1.57	42%
	0.5 μg 60-70S RNA	Poly U + 0.1 μg Oligo T	1.46	40%
Control	0.5 μg 60-70S RNA		3.7	100%
	0.5 μg 60-70S RNA	+ 0.1 μg Oligo T	10.6	290%

6.5 μg of 60-70S ^{32}P-RNA was hybridized to 15 μg of ^{3}H-Poly U. Both components were heated in 0.01 M Tris (pH 7.4) and 0.25 NaCl to 48 °C in a water bath and allowed to cool down overnight. The assay then was layered on a gradient (10—25% sucrose), centrifuged at 64,000 rpm, 45 min, 20 °C) and the 60-70S RNA peak separated; 0.3 μg of ^{3}H Poly U (= 4.5% of the amount of the RNA) was hybridized to the 60-70S RNA.

These results may imply that RSV RNA contains two kinds of poly A regions. One kind can function as a DNA initiation site on native RNA; perhaps because the poly A is in juxtaposition to primer RNA. This fraction of poly A can be masked by poly U, and this would explain the inhibitory effect of the hybridized poly U. The other kind of poly A in RSV RNA may be activated for initiation of DNA synthesis only in the presence of Oligo T. This would explain why Oligo T increases the template activity of 60-70S RNA 2—3-fold. This raises the question: Is poly A (or part of it) transcribed, or only used as an initiation recognition signal?

Transcription of Poly A

A nearest neighbor analysis of the *in vitro* synthesized DNA was performed. In this experiment a radioactive phosphate of the 5′ thymidyl end is transferred to the 3′ end of its next neighbor nucleotide dA, dC, or dG by micrococcus nuclease hydrolysis; thus telling us the frequency of neighbor sequences of bases dA, dC, or dG to dT within the DNA [32].

Table 3 shows the results of an *in vitro* experiment on the kinetics of DNA synthesis after digestion of the DNA by nucleases, and electrophoresis of the monophosphate digestion products.

Table 3. Nearest neighbor analysis of *in vitro* synthesized DNA

– Oligo T cpm ^{32}p					+ Oligo T cpm ^{32}p			
Time of incubation	dC_pT	dA_pT	dG_pT	T_pT	dC_pT	dA_pT	dG_pT	T_pT
10 min	98	85	76	215	135	115	130	1900
30 min	205	195	175	390				
120 min	1040	950	865	1950	800	745	730	9200

The standard assay as in Table 1 was incubated for 2 hrs (using (4×10^{-5} M) α-^{32}P-TTP (0.3 Ci/mmole) instead of ^{3}H-TTP). The digestion conditions were as follows: The DNA-product was freed from unincorporated labeled TTP by four-fold TCA precipitation. The DNA was digested by 170 U micrococcal nuclease for 50 min 37 °C, and subsequently digested by 0.17 U splen phosphodiesterase. Electrophoresis was for 3 hrs at 1500 V on Whatman 3 MM paper. The radioactive spots were identified by parallel migrating deoxyribonucleoside-monophosphates and counted in a scintillation counter.

About 80% of the XpT sequences were present as TpT sequences in DNA made on 70S RNA in the presence of Oligo T. However, DNA produced on native 70S RNA (no Oligo T) also contains TpT sequences, though in a much lower amount; 40% of the XpT sequences were TpT sequences and 20% for each dApT, dCpT, dGpT. This is evidence that at least part of the A rich regions of native 70S RNA are transcribed to poly T. Moreover, the results suggest that Oligo T specifically primes transcription of A rich sequences of 60-70S RSV RNA.

Another indication that poly A is transcribed is the finding that omission of TTP in the polymerase assay abolishes DNA synthesis almost completely. Omission of dATP, dCTP, and dGTP however, only reduces "DNA" synthesis to 8% of TMP incorporation (acid insoluble) compared to 100% TMP incorporation in the presence of all four DNA precursors (Table 4). This TMP incorporation probably represents poly T synthesis on natural primers. In the presence of Oligo T, poly T synthesis is even 30—40% of the DNA synthesis under normal conditions (4 nucleotides).

In order to establish that this poly T synthesis is not generated by artificial addition of TMP to Oligo T primer, we also used Oligo dC as primer. Sixteen percent TMP is incorporated compared to 100% in the presence of all four precursors (the weaker binding of Oligo C to poly A compared to the strong Oligo T-poly A binding may cause the lower synthesis of poly T).

Table 4. Poly-T synthesis

Substrate present	Oligo-nucleotide	pmole incorp./60 min TMP	dCMP	
{dA, dC, dG [a] TTP-^{3}H		4.15		100%
TTP-^{3}H only		0.33		8%
{dA, dC, dG [a] TTP-^{3}H	Oligo T	21.0		100%
TTP-^{3}H only	Oligo T	8.1		39%
{dA, dC, dG [a] TTP-^{3}H	Oligo dC	13.2		100%
TTP-^{3}H only	Oligo dC	2.1		16%
{dA, dG, T [a] dCTP-^{3}H			3.9	100%
dCTP-^{3}H only			0.82	2.1%
{dA, dG, T [a] dCTP-^{3}H	Oligo T		10.0	100%
dCTP-^{3}H only	Oligo T		0.24	2.4%

[a] i. e. triphosphates of indicated nucleotides
Standard assay was incubated with indicated substrates and oligonucleotides.

The Size of Poly T

The size of poly T produced in the presence of Oligo T is about 2-4S, according to sucrose gradient centrifugation with 4S t-RNA as marker (Fig. 2). That reflects a fairly quantitative transcription of poly A regions, and suggests furthermore that Oligo T at the concentrations used does not completely cover the poly A regions of 60-70S RSV RNA.

Discussion

Whether this demonstrated *in vitro* transcription of poly A to poly T is analogous to *in vivo* transcription is not yet known. If, however, replication of RNA takes place in the postulated pathway via a DNA intermediate, it appears to be necessary to transcribe the A rich clusters into poly T within the DNA in order to transcribe

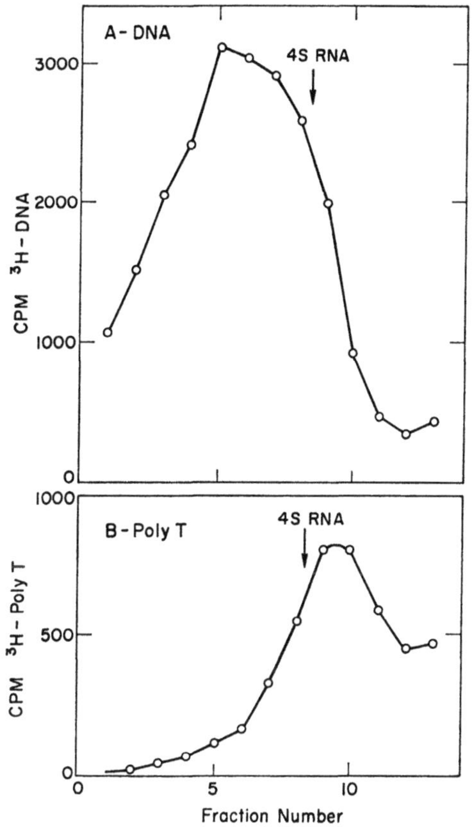

Fig. 2. Sucrose gradient sedimentation of *in vitro* DNA and poly T produced *in vitro* using standard assay that contained 0.1 μg Oligo T and in (A) all four deoxynucleoside triphosphates and in (B) only TTP-^{3}H as substrate. Centrifugation was 64,000 rpm, 11 hrs. 20 °C in 10—25% sucrose gradient containing 0.1% SDS

it properly back to the progeny RNA. The search for vial DNA may be facilitated by looking for poly T in the DNA of transformed cells. — Though the *in vitro* experiments with the viral DNA polymerase do not give us final proof of the provirus hypothesis, at least the possibility of transcription from RNA to DNA using an endogenous viral enzyme and viral RNA is now demonstrated.

In this context the question is often raised: Whether the virus polymerase is really virus-specific, since RNA dependent DNA polymerase activity is also found in uninfected cells [33, 34]. Firstly, it is possible that this cellular enzyme(s) has different specificity — recent results show structural and serological behavior different from the viral enzyme [34]. Secondly, some pages above we left the question unanswered why hybridization experiments between viral RNA and cellular DNA exhibit little if any difference between uninfected and infected cells.

Recent results, in particular the induction of non-transforming RNA tumor viruses in "virus free" animal cells by chemical agents or radiation [35 b], are compatible with the idea that genetic material of RNA tumor viruses already *pre-exists* in all animal cells, integrated into cellular DNA. The oncogene-hypothesis by HUEBNER [35], and the protovirus hypothesis by TEMIN [36] which both predicted those findings, say that virus genes and/or oncogens are integrated into animal DNA but normally not expressed. Therefore viruses are not produced, nor is any oncogenic behavior exhibited. It is, however, conceivable that only synthesis of "harmful" oncogene products is turned off and "harmless" gene functions like the viral "reverse transcriptase" are expressed.

I do not intend to go into a discussion about this very recent and fascinating problem. It is to suppose that there is ubiquity of the potential for malignant transformation of animal cells in the form of genetic information of RNA tumor viruses.

"Do not interfere with a pending trial" is an old proverb of the Romans. Thus a paper about the replication of RNA tumor viruses written some years later may end with rather different conclusions.

Summary

Regarding the RNA dependent DNA polymerase of RSV there are some properties of the enzyme that favor its crucial role in the virus replication and some that do not support this concept. Recent observations on the behaviour of RNA of the Rous sarcoma lead up to a hypothetical model of this RNA used as template for DNA synthesis. An *in vitro* transcription of poly A to poly T is suggested. The results are discussed in connection with recent hypothesis in molecular biology including the oncogene and the protovirus hypothesis.

Acknowledgment

I thank Dr. PETER DUESBERG for his excellent advice and encouragement. The editorial assistance of JAN MAISEL is gratefully acknowledged.

This investigation was supported by U. S. Public Health Service Research Grant CA 11426 from the National Cancer Institute, and in part by Cancer Research Funds from the University of California, and Contract No. 71-2173 within the special Virus-Cancer Program of the National Cancer Institute, NIH, PHS, and a Deutsche Forschungs-Gemeinschaft fellowship.

References

1. TEMIN, H. M.: Virology **20**, 577 (1963).
2. BADER, J. P.: Virology **40**, 494 (1970).
3. DUESBERG, P. H., VOGT, P.: Proc. nat. Acad. Sci. (Wash.) **64**, 939 (1969).
4. BADER, J. P., BADER, A. V.: Proc. nat. Acad. Sci. (Wash.) **67**, 843 (1970).
5. RUBIN, H., TEMIN, H. M.: Virology **7**, 75 (1959).
6. TEMIN, H. M.: Virology **23**, 486 (1964).
7. BADER, J. P.: Virology **26**, 253 (1965).
8. TEMIN, H. M.: Proc. nat. Acad. Sci. (Wash.) **52**, 323 (1964).
9. WOLLMANN, R. L., KIRSTEN, W. H.: J. Virol. **3**, 1241 (1968).
10. BALUDA, M. A., NAYAK, D. P.: Proc. nat. Acad. Sci. (Wash.) **66**, 329 (1970).
11. ROSENTHAL, P. N., ROBINSON, H. J., ROBINSON, W. S., HANAFUSA, T., HANAFUSA, H.: Proc. nat. Acad. Sci. (Wash.) **68**, 2336 (1971).
12. GELB, L. D., AARONSON, S. A., MARTIN, M.: Science **172**, 1353 (1971).

13a. VARMUS, H. E., LEVINSON, W. E., BISHOP, J. M.: Nature (Lond.) New Biol. **233**, 19 (1971).
13b. LEONG, J. A., GARAPIN, A. C., JACKSON, N., FANSHIER, L., LEVINSON, W., BISHOP, J. M.: J. Virol. 1972 (submitted).
14. TEMIN, H. M., MIZUTANI, S.: Nature (Lond.) **266**, 1211 (1970).
15. BALTIMORE, D.: Nature (Lond.) **226**, 1209 (1970).
16. SPIEGELMAN, S. *et al.*: Nature (Lond.) **227**, 563 (1970).
17. GALLO, R., YANG, S. S., TING, R. C.: Nature (Lond.) **228**, 927 (1970).
18. TEMIN, H. M.: Ann. Rev. Microbiol. **25**, 609 (1971).
19. DUESBERG, P. H., CANAANI, E.: Virology **42**, 783 (1970).
20. DUESBERG, P. H., v. D. HELM, K., CANAANI, E.: Proc. nat. Acad. Sci. (Wash.) **68**, 747 (1971).
21. DUESBERG, P. H., v. D. HELM, K., CANAANI, E.: Proc. nat. Acad. Sci. (Wash.) **68**, 2505 (1971).
22. HURWITZ, J., LEIS, J. P.: J. Virol. **9**, 116 (1972).
23. LEIS, J. P., HURWITZ, J.: J. Virol. **9**, 130 (1972).
24. VERMA, I. M., MEUTH, N. L., BROMFELD, E., MANLY, K. F., BALTIMORE, D.: Nature (Lond.) New Biol. **233**, 131 (1971).
25. ROBINSON, W. S., PITKÄNEN, A., RUBIN, H.: Proc. nat. Acad. Sci. (Wash.) **54**, 137 (1965).
26. DUESBERG, P. H.: Proc. nat. Acad. Sci. (Wash.) **60**, 1511 (1968).
27. DUESBERG, P. H., VOGT, P.: Proc. nat. Acad. Sci. (Wash.) **67**, 1673 (1970).
28. ERIKSON, R. L., ERIKSON, E.: J. Virol. **8**, 254 (1971).
29. LAI, M., DUESBERG, P. H.: Nature (Lond.) **235**, 383 (1972).
30. STEINER, R., BEERS, R.: Polynucleotides. New York: Elsevier 1961.
31. v. D. HELM, K., unpublished results.
32. JOSSE, J., KAISER, A. D., KORNBERG, A.: J. biol. Chem. **236**, 864 (1961).
33. SCOLNIK, E. M., AARONSON, S. A., TODARO, G., PARKS, W.: Nature (Lond.) **229**, 318 (1971).
34. ROSS, J., SCOLNIK, E. M., TODARO, G., AARONSON, S. A.: Nature (Lond.) New Biology **231**, 163 (1971).
35a. HUEBNER, R. T., TODARO, G.: Proc. nat. Acad. Sci. (Wash.) **64**, 1087 (1969).
35b. TODARO, G., HUEBNER, R. T.: Proc. nat. Acad. Sci. (Wash.) **69**, 1009 (1972).
36. TEMIN, H.: J. nat. Cancer Inst. **46**, III (1971).
37. CANAANI, E., DUESBERG, P. H.: J. Virol. **10**, 23 (1972).

Differentiation of Tumor Cells*

Induction of Erythrocyte Membrane-Specific Antigens in Friend Leukemia Cells

H. SUGANO, M. FURUSAWA, T. KAWAGUCHI, and Y. IKAWA

Introduction

It was believed for a long time, in both experimental and clinical fields that every cancer had its own malignancy and progressed into a more malignant state after a certain period. In other words, the cancer phenotype was stable and if it changed, it progressed only towards a more malignant state. Cancerization was thought to be irreversible. Ten years ago, YOSHIDA *et al.* [43] concluded that an irreversible change in a benign direction can very rarely occur in tumor cells. In viral carcinogenesis *in vitro*, MACPHERSON [25] demonstrated a revertant colony derived from cloned transformed cells. BRAUN [4] discussed the reversal of tumor growth from the viewpoint of gene regulation. Recently, SUGIMURA [40] also stressed a certain phenotypic change of a tumor as "decarcinogenesis" in his enzymic study of tumors. In the clinical field, as EVERSON and COLE [6] noted, spontaneous regression of human cancer definitely occurs.

Regarding these, it is apparent that the cancer phenotype can be unstable and sometimes changes into a less malignant state or towards the normal condition. This phenomenon is called reversion of tumor cells, tumor reversal, or differentiation of tumor cells. Reversion of tumor cells or tumor reversal usually implies that the tumor cells return towards a normal state and show loss of or decline in their transplantability, while differentiation or maturation of tumor cells indicates the appearance of the phenotype which is characteristic of the normal mother tissue.

Past reports of reversion of tumor cells may be summarized as follows:

1. Reversion of human tumors: Reversions of neuroblastoma and Grawitz tumor are most prominent, followed by melanoma and chorioepithelioma [6]. The high antigenicity of these tumors probably plays an important role in their reversion.

2. Reversion of transplantable tumors: YOSHIDA *et al.* [43], using immunologically sensitized rats, produced variants of Yoshida sarcoma which were much less malignant than the original Yoshida sarcoma. The isozyme pattern of hexokinase

---

* This study was partly supported by a Grant-in-Aid from the Ministry of Education, and the Ministry of Health and Welfare, Government of Japan.

We thank Mr. T. NASHIRO for his skilful assistance in electron microscopy.

in these variant tumor cells changed and was similar to that of Morris hepatoma and normal liver [33, 40].

3. Natural reversion of tumor cells cultured *in vitro:* There are many reports of natural reversion of tumor cells being induced by chemicals and viruses. During a long-term culture period, the transplantability of tumor cells into susceptible normal animals decreased gradually and finally disappeared.

4. Artificial reversion of tumor cells cultured *in vitro:* Cultured cells have been observed to change their transplantability as a result of treatment with chemical substances such as 4-nitroquinolin 1-oxide (4NQO) [24], 5-bromodeoxyuridine (BudR) [36], Actinomycin-D [2], N-nitrosomethylurea (NMU) [31], etc.

5. Reversion of cells by cell hybridization: A hybrid cell, consisting of a tumor cell and a normal cell sometimes showed reduction in transplantability [16]. The degree of reduction in transplantability depended on the normal cell used as a component of the hybrid cell.

6. Transient differentiation of cultured tumor cells: The phenotypic changes observed in the above-mentioned revertants, except the human tumors, are considered to be permanent reversions. In these cases, a certain change of phenotype occurred in the tumor cell and a new character became stable. In other cases, a temporary reversion of tumor cells was observed during treatment with substances like Concanavalin-A (Con A) [5], BudR [30, 35], dibutyryl-AMP, cyclic-AMP [21], and others.

7. Differentiation of cultured cells caused by an inducer: A conditioned medium, obtained from a culture medium in which spleen cells and fibroblasts were grown, was found to be useful for the induction of differentiation in granulocytic leukemia [17]. Differentiation of Stansly leukemia cells and Friend cells in the peritoneal cavity [11, 37] was also observed by a diffusion chamber technique. Therefore, it is suggested that some factor or factors present in the body may induce the reversion or differentiation of tumor cells.

In order to examine tumor reversion, it is important to select a marker which is usually a characteristic feature of the cell morphology, chromosome analysis, biochemical activity, isozyme pattern, cell growth, transplantability, or antigenicity. Cell agglutination properties are also useful. In the body, each tissue cell has its own marker. Tumor cells sometimes preserve the markers of the original tissue, but often they show some markers characteristic of other organs. Deviation of the markers is a characteristic feature of the tumor which may be explained by the switch-on and -off theory of gene expression. If a marker is highly specific, reversion may be clearly demonstrated. Acetylcholinesterase activity [3, 22] in neuroblastoma cells, and production of melanin pigment and tyrosinase activity in melanoma cells [36] are such examples. Erythroid leukemia cells also have excellent markers, hemoglobin syntheses and erythrocyte membrane-specific antigens.

We have been studying leukemogenesis and differentiation of Friend leukemia, and the differentiation of Friend leukemia cells will be described in the present article.

Differentiation of Friend Leukemia Cells

Friend leukemia, first described by FRIEND [7], was induced by the Friend leukemia virus (FLV) in Swiss mice. The mice with Friend leukemia showed characteristic splenomegaly, containing large leukemia cells (hereafter referred to as Friend cells) which were erythroid in nature. FRIEND *et al.* [8, 26, 29] clearly demonstrated erythroid differentiation of Friend cells by the soft agar technique.

Ascitic Friend leukemia and cultured Friend cells, which originated from a spleen colony induced by FLV in a male DDD mouse [18, 19] were maintained in our laboratory for 4 years. These cells, which are also erythroid, clearly demonstrated heme synthesis [32] and globin synthesis [23].

An erythroid tumor cell, such as a Friend cell, should be a very good model for examining the differentiation of a tumor cell for the following reasons.

1. There are definite markers in the erythroid cell for example hemoglobin synthesis and erythrocyte membrane-specific antigens (see the following chapter).

2. The step of differentiation and the kinetics of erythroblasts are well known in normal hematopoiesis *in vivo*.

3. Certain substances, e.g. Erythropoietin and Vitamin B_{12}, give specific effects on the cells of erythroid series.

4. A Friend cell carries the FLV genome. This is interesting in relation to the expression of the viral genome in differentiation of Friend cells. If the viral genome could be eliminated from a Friend cell, the cell could possibly differentiate into an erythrocyte.

Conditions and substances which enhance erythroid differentiation of Friend cells *in vivo* and *in vitro* were examined extensively by using the fluorescein antibody technique for erythrocyte membrane-specific antigens as the characteristic marker of an erythroid cell.

Mouse Erythrocyte Membrane-specific Antigens (MEM-Antigens), as a Marker of an Erythroid Cell

FURUSAWA and ADACHI [1, 10] purified two kinds of specific membrane proteins of normal mouse erythrocytes and obtained 'anti-A serum', which contained an erythrocyte membrane-specific antibody, by immunizing guinea pigs with the 'aqueous phase' of a butanol fraction of the membrane proteins. Fluorescein isothiocyanate (FITC)-conjugated anti-A serum was used to stain specifically cells of the erythroid series of a mouse, from proerythroblasts to erythrocytes. The cells were stained by the conjugated antibodies after fixation with cold acetone and examined with a fluorescence microscope using Orsen's FITC Interference Filter. The intensity of fluorescence of the erythroid cells varied and depended on their degree of maturation in the erythroid series i.e. proerythroblasts were slightly and erythrocytes strongly stained. Thus the synthesis of erythrocyte membrane-specific antigens was shown to parallel the differentiation of the erythroid series. An erythroid cell can therefore be specifically identified by using this conjugated antibody technique.

Erythrocytes of rats and hamsters, both golden and Chinese hamsters, were also slightly stained by the conjugated antibodies. Therefore, these specific antigens are distributed not only in mouse erythrocytes but also to a lesser extent in the erythrocytes of *Myomorpha* [12].

Hereafter, the antigens obtained from the mouse erythrocytes will be referred to as mouse erythrocyte membrane-specific antigens (MEM-antigens).

Distribution of MEM-Antigens in the Friend Cells

The conjugated antibodies clearly stained the primary Friend cells in the spleen of DDD mice with FLV-induced Friend disease. The cytoplasm of all the Friend cells was stained diffusely [20]. This result gave us a conclusive evidence of the erythroid nature of the Friend cells, and indicated that maturation was at the level of proerythroblasts.

Cultured Friend cells (designated TSFAT-3-C1-1) grew well in suspension culture. The generation time of the cells was approximately 20 hr and the modal number of chromosomes per cell was 75. The cell morphology was either similar to that of proerythroblasts or basophilic erythroblasts. The cell diameter was 20 μ in the cells of the former and 15 μ in the latter.

The cultured cells were very slightly positive to conjugated antibody staining 24 hr after the cells had been newly seeded (Fig. 1). The cells were still falsely positive on the 2nd and 3rd days after the medium change; after the 4th day, all the cells became completely negative [38].

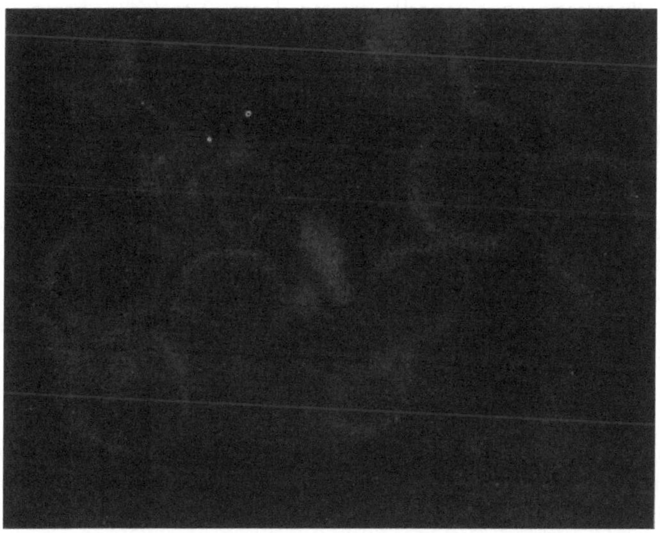

Fig. 1. Fluorescein-conjugated antibody staining of nontreated Friend cells cultured *in vitro*. The cells show a very slight fluorescence in the cytoplasm. ×2,000

It is therefore clear that the MEM-antigens were strongly produced in the primary Friend cells when Friend disease occurred *in vivo*. After long-term culture, most of the Friend cells lost the power to synthesize MEM-antigens, but still maintained some slight erythrocytic gene expression.

Induction of MEM-Antigens in the Friend Cells

1. *In vivo* Study: Cells Cultured in the Peritoneal Cavity of Mice Syngeneic to the Friend Cells

The cultured Friend cells grew well in the peritoneal cavity of DDD mice syngeneic to Friend cells and easily became an ascitic form. Ascitic Friend cells could possibly undergo erythroid maturation in the peritoneal cavity, but these cells were completely negative to membrane-specific antibody staining. It was postulated from this result that if erythroid maturation had occurred in a few cells, these cells might have been eliminated by an overwhelming majority of other Friend cells. Therefore, a diffusion chamber technique was used to study a small number of Friend cells. The cells cultured in a diffusion chamber clearly demonstrated an erythrocytic expression [11, 13].

The Friend cells of TSFAT-3-C1-1 line, approximately 5×10^4 or 2×10^5 cells, were placed in a diffusion chamber, securely sealed with Millipore membrane pads (0.45 μ pore size) and cultured in the peritoneal cavity of DDD mice for 4 to 9 days.

The results from each chamber were not always the same. Generally, the proportion of smaller cells was larger than had been found in the original culture. In the most cases, the predominant portion was occupied by the cells of 10 to 15 μ in diameter, resembling basophilic or polychromophilic erythroblasts. In some cases (5 to 20 chambers), small anucleate, erythrocyte-like corpuscles were seen. Conjugated antibody staining revealed that the tumor cells showed a positive reaction. The proportion of fluorescein-positive cells ranged from 2 to 90%, being 20—30% in most cases, with the smaller cells tending to show stronger fluorescence than larger ones. Some anucleated erythrocyte-like cells fluoresced as strongly as normal erythrocytes. Similar control experiments were carried out using cultured lymphoma cells, induced by Moloney leukemia virus in a mouse, and a completely negative result was obtained.

Electron photomicrographs of the cells cultured in chambers revealed a great number of virus particles in cytoplasmic vacuoles, while only a few virus particles were observed in the non-treated Friend cells. During these experiments, marked splenomegaly was noted in most of the mice in which the diffusion chambers had been placed. The splenomegaly of mice in this experiment was larger than that of the mice in which Friend cells (1×10^8 cells) were transplanted intraperitoneally as a routine transplantation. It is therefore suggested that production of virus particles was greatly exaggerated in the Friend cells cultured in a diffusion chamber.

It was concluded from this experiment that Friend cells were able to enhance the erythrocytic expression *in vivo*, and it is suggested that there is a factor in the body which enhances erythrocytic maturation.

2. *In vivo* Study: The Cells Cultured in the Peritoneal Cavity of Rats Allogeneic to Friend Cells

It was assumed that erythrocytic expression of Friend cells might be accelerated in an animal allogeneic to the cell. Therefore, a similar experiment was carried out with rats [39]. Friend cells (2×10^5) were placed in diffusion chambers sealed with Millipore membranes and cultured in the peritoneal cavity of male Donryu rats for 2 to 7 days. The cells in each chamber gave almost the same results. Most of the cells gradually became smaller and resembled mature erythroblasts, and almost all the cells were strongly positive to erythrocyte-specific antibody staining. The intensity of fluorescence of the cells increased gradually during the culture and its maximum was on the 4th day of culture. After the 5th day the cells became rapidly damaged until (on the 7th day) most of the cells showed complete degeneration.

Many virus particles were observed by electron microscopy in the vacuoles which were usually located to one side of the cytoplasm of the cell. The shape of the virus particles, which consisted in this experiment of both mature and immature type-C particles was much more irregular than those found in nontreated Friend cells (Fig. 2). Splenomegaly was not observed in the rats into which the diffusion chambers had been placed.

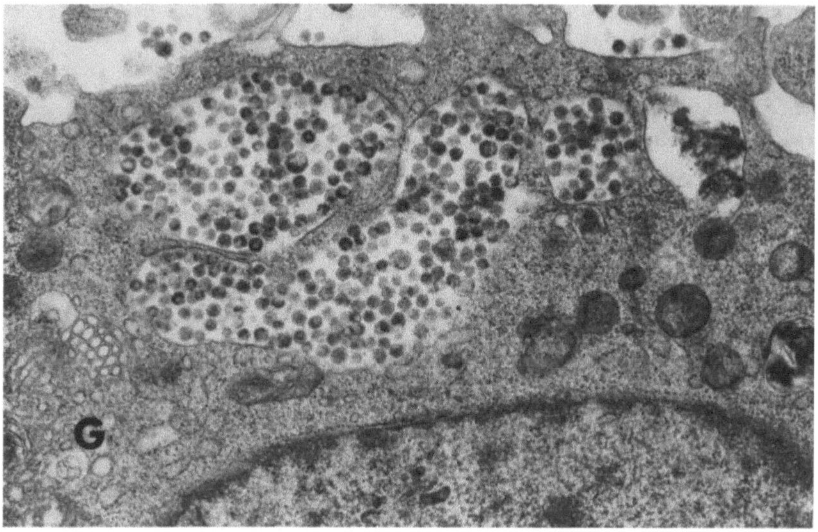

Fig. 2. Electron micrograph of a Friend cell cultured for 5 days in a diffusion chamber in the peritoneal cavity of a rat, allogeneic to the Friend cell. Numerous type-C virus particles can be observed in the vacuoles which are located near the Golgi apparatus (G). Virus particles are irregular in size and shape. ×22,000

This experiment shows that erythrocytic expression is greatly exaggerated in an allogeneic animal. In both mice and rats the diffusion chamber became filled with a gelatinous material in which Friend cells were enclosed. It is possible that the special environmental conditions within a chamber may have been sufficient in themselves to cause erythrocytic differentiation, without the need to postulate the existence of an external factor which could enhance the maturation.

3. *In vitro* Experiments

In order to analyze the mechanism involved in maturation of Friend cells, various substances and conditions which enhance erythrocytic expression *in vitro* were studied, including the use of dimethyl sulfoxide (DMSO) which was first applied by Friend *et al.* [9, 34].

The cells were seeded into 70-mm culture bottles at the concentration of 1×10^5 cells/ml of fresh medium and, at the same time, various substances diluted to an appropriate concentration were added. On the 3rd day, a fresh medium containing the same concentration of the substances was added. On the 2nd and 4th days after the treatment, the cells were centrifuged and prepared for fluorescein-conjugated antibody staining, Giemsa staining, and electron microscopy. The most effective concentration of each substance for erythrocytic expression was determined and the effective range was also checked. The fluorescein-conjugated antibody staining was used as the main technique in this experiment [38]. The results obtained in the experiments were as follows:

a) **Inhibitors of DNA, RNA, and Protein Synthesis.** As Table 1 shows, all the inhibitors of DNA synthesis, cytosine arabinoside (ara-C), 5-fluorodeoxyuridine (FudR), and N-hydroxyurea, moderately to markedly increased the erythrocyte-specific antibody staining, with ara-C being the most effective (Fig. 3). Under the influence of these substances the cells increased in size becoming twice as large as the control Friend cells. With the Giemsa staining, the cytoplasm and the surface of the

Table 1. Substances enhancing MEM-specific antigens

	Effect	Most effective doses	Range
Ara-C	(+++)	1×10^{-6} M	$1\times10^{-8}-1\times10^{-5}$ M
FudR	(++)	1×10^{-6} M	$1\times10^{-7}-1\times10^{-5}$ M
Hydroxyurea	(++)	6.5×10^{-4} M	$1\times10^{-7}-1\times10^{-4}$ M
BudR	(−)		$1\times10^{-7}-1\times10^{-3}$ M
Actinomycin D	(−)		0.5 −50.0 μg/ml
Puromycin	(−)		0.01− 0.1 μg/ml
Cycloheximide	(−)		0.1 − 1.0 μg/ml
X-ray irradiation	(−)		200−900 r

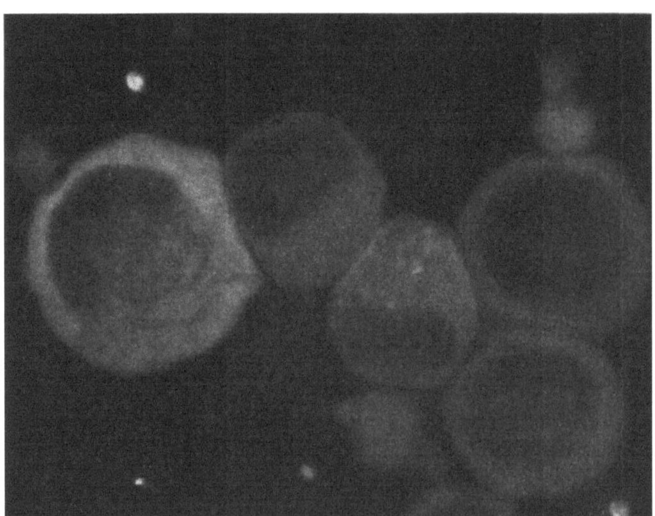

Fig. 3. Fluorescein-conjugated antibody staining of Friend cells treated with cytosin arabinoside (1×10^{-6} M) for 4 days. The cytoplasm of the enlarged Friend cells is diffusely stained. The cells became larger. ×2,000

cells were diffusely and strongly stained respectively, while the nucleus remained unstained. In these cases the production of MEM-antigens was already markedly enhanced on the 2nd day. On the other hand, the cells treated with 5-bromodeoxyuridine (BudR) [35], Actinomycin-D, Puromycin, and Cycloheximide did not stain. X-Ray irradiation was also ineffective. The cells became smaller with all substances except BudR, which caused no change in size. It was expected that inhibitors of DNA synthesis might be effective and inhibitors of RNA and protein synthesis not effective, because protein synthesis is closely related to the cell cycle. When cell growth stops, maturation occurs in most cases. SCHUBERT and JACOB [35] clearly demonstrated that BudR accelerated the differentiation of neuroblastoma *in vitro,* but no such effect was observed in our experiments.

b) Anticancer Agents. As indicated in Table 2, all the anticancer agents examined enhanced erythrocytic expression; Bleomycin [41], ara-C, and Mitomycin-C (MMC) were moderately to markedly effective while nitrogen mustard, Vincristine, and 5-fluorouracil (5-FU) were only slightly effective. The size of the cells increased to twice that of the non-treated cells, and their cytoplasm was diffusely and strongly fluorescent often accompanied by numerous fine dots which were intensely fluorescent. Bleomycin gave the most intense fluorescence (Fig. 4). In these cases, the synthesis of erythrocyte-specific antigens was already clearly enhanced by the 2nd day.

Table 2. Substances enhancing MEM-specific antigens

	Effect	Most effective doses	Range
Bleomycin	(+++)	3.0 μg/ml	0.1–50.0 μg/ml
Ara-C	(+++)	1×10^{-6} M	1×10^{-8}–1×10^{-5} M
MMC	(++)	1.0 μg/ml	0.1–5.0 μg/ml
Nitrogen mustard	(+)	1×10^{-6} M	1×10^{-7}–1×10^{-5} M
Vincristine	(+)	1×10^{-9} M	1×10^{-10}–1×10^{-9} M
5-FU	(+)	1×10^{-5} M	1×10^{-6}–1×10^{-5} M

It is interesting that anticancer agents not only killed the cancer cells but also enhanced the maturation of tumor cells.

c) Erythropoietin, Vitamin B_{12}, and Cyclic AMP. Erythropoietin (Ep) and vitamin B_{12} (VB_{12}) have specific effects on erythropoiesis. Cyclic dibutyryl-AMP, $(But)_2$-cAMP, shows various effects on the cell and induces morphological differentiation of tumor cells [21]. The effect of these substances, either singly or in combination, on Friend cells is shown in Table 3.

Ep was shown to be slightly effective in enhancing erythrocyte expression while VB_{12} and $(But)_2$-cAMP were ineffective. A combination of two of these three substances gave moderate and diffuse fluorescence. The cells grew well and became slightly smaller, the intensity of fluorescence gradually increasing after treatment. It is postulated that a stem cell, the erythropoietin-reacting cell (ERc), differentiates into a proerythroblast under the influence of Ep. In this experiment, Ep was effective on Friend cells while VB_{12} was not effective. This may indicate that the Friend cells cultured *in vitro* stop at the level of ERc of stem cells. It is suggested that

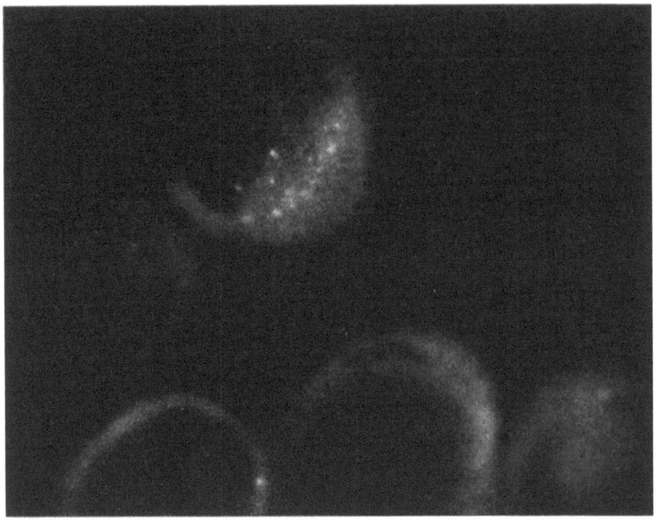

Fig. 4. Fluorescein-conjugated antibody staining of Friend cells treated with Bleomycin (3.0 μg/ml) for 4 days. The cells became larger. The cytoplasm stained diffusely and several bright dots can be seen in some instances. ×2,000

erythrocytic maturation of the cell induced by a combination of two of the three substances is very similar to normal erythroid maturation.

d) Substances Effective on the Cell Surface. The results obtained with the substances which are mainly effective on the cell surface are indicated in Table 4. The Friend cells treated with nonionic detergents, Tween 80 and Nonidet (Sodium lauryl sulfate), were almost negative to conjugated antibody staining. An extract of a root of *Phytolacca americana* (PA) acts similarly to Phytohemagglutinin (PHA) in causing blastic transformation of human lymphocytes and hemagglutination [42]. PA, both trypsinized and non-trypsinized, was ineffective in enhancing MEM-antigens. Con-A was also ineffective while trypsinized Con-A was slightly effective. Burger *et al.* [5] and Sachs *et al.* [28] stressed the alteration of the tumor cell surfaces when reversion was induced with Con-A. So far as the present experiments are concerned, the results may suggest that the synthesis of erythrocyte-specific antigens is not closely related to the alteration of the cell surface.

Table 3. Substances enhancing MEM-specific antigens

	Effect	Most effective doses	Range
Erythropoietin	(+)	0.2 U	0.02 – 0.2 U
Vitamin B_{12}	(−)		0.1 – 5.0 μg/ml
$(But)_2$-cAMP	(−)		0.1 – 100.0 μg/ml
Ep + $(But)_2$-cAMP	(++)	0.2 U + 100 μg	
Ep + VB_{12}	(++)	0.2 U + 5.0 μg	
VB_{12} + $(But)_2$-cAMP	(++)	5.0 μg + 100.0 μg	

Table 4. Substances enhancing MEM-specific antigens

	Effect	Most effective doses	Range
Tween 80	(±)	0.5%	
Nonidet	(−)		0.001 – 0.01%
PA [a]	(−)		0.4 – 40.0 μg/ml
Concanavalin A	(−)		10.0 – 50.0 μg/ml
Trypsinized-Con A	(+)	100.0 μg/ml	20.0 – 200.0 μg/ml

[a] Extract of the root of *Phytolacca americana*.

e) Other Substances and Conditions. The results obtained from cells treated with other substances and under other conditions are indicated in Table 5. FRIEND *et al.* [9, 34] reported most striking evidence of the erythroid maturation of Friend cells using dimethyl sulfoxide (DMSO). In our experiments, DMSO was one of the most interesting substances which induced erythroid maturation of the Friend cells. The Friend cells treated with DMSO gave intense fluorescence with conjugated antibody staining which became prominent on the 4th day (Fig. 5). The cytoplasm of the cells was diffusely stained, accompanied by rather large dots markedly positive to the fluorescent-antibody. These dots were usually observed in the submembranous area and sometimes in the perinuclear area. In some instances, a bright dot appeared in the perinuclear area, apparently in the Golgi area, and enlarged after treatment. As SATO *et al.* [34] reported, many virus particles were observed electron microscopically in the vacuoles of the cytoplasm. It is suggested that the brightly stained spots correspond to the virus-containing vacuoles. The cells became gradually smaller and resembled mature erythroblasts.

N-dimethyl-rifampicin, an inhibitor of the reverse transcriptase of RNA-oncogenic viruses [14, 15], and its derivative Rifamide, were effective in induction of MEM-antigens. After staining, numerous bright dots appeared in the cytoplasm of the Friend cells treated with N-dimethyl-rifampicin (Fig. 6). Fluorescence of the

Table 5. Substances and culture conditions enhancing MEM-specific antigens

	Effect	Most effective doses	Range
DMSO	(+++)	2.0%	0.5 – 5.0%
N-dimethyl-rifampicin	(+++)	100.0 μg/ml	50.0 – 200.0 μg/ml
Rifamide	(++)	100.0 μg/ml	50.0 – 200.0 μg/ml
Glycerin	(++)	5%	2.0 – 10.0%
Cultured			
at 32 °C	(+)		
without serum	(+)		
add. excess fetal calf serum	(−)		

cells became most prominent on the 4th day and the cells became slightly smaller. Electron photomicrographs revealed a few virus particles in the endoplasmic reticulum of the cytoplasm.

Glycerin was moderately effective in inducing the production of MEM-antigens and the cells became slightly larger. The cells cultured at 32° C and those cultured

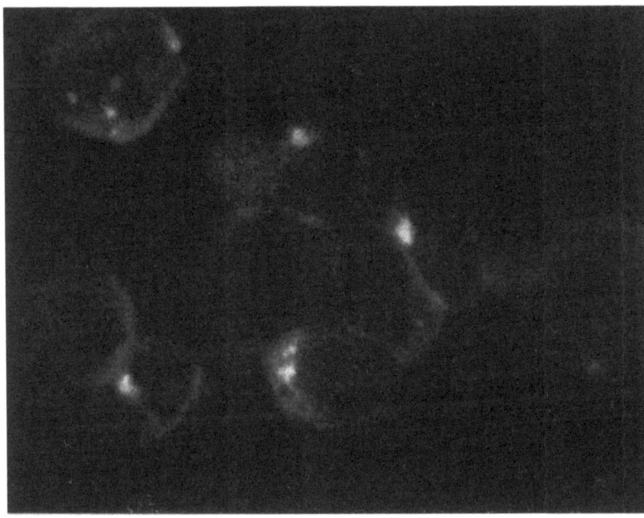

Fig. 5. Fluorescein-conjugated antibody staining of Friend cells treated with 2% DMSO for 5 days. Rather large clearly fluorescent dots in the cytoplasm are characteristic of this treatment. The cells became smaller. ×2,000

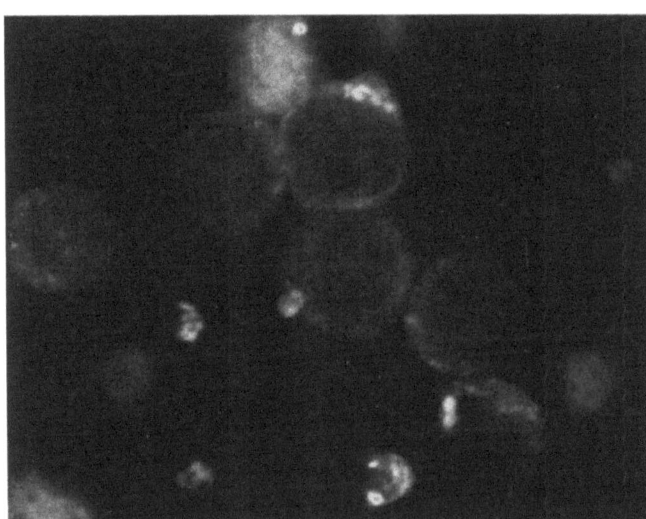

Fig. 6. Fluorescein-conjugated antibody staining of Friend cells treated with N-dimethylrifampicin (100 μg/ml) for 4 days. The cytoplasm stained diffusely, but bright dots can also be seen. The cells became slightly smaller. ×2,000

in a medium without calf serum gave a slight fluorescence, while the cells cultured in a medium containing excess fetal calf serum were ineffective in producing the antigens.

Discussion

1. Leukemogenesis and Differentiation

The origin of Friend cells seems to be from stem cells and immature erythroblasts. The Friend cells in the original mouse were positive to conjugated antibody staining [20] and it is considered that these Friend cells are already erythrocyte-directed cells in which differentiation has stopped at the level of proerythroblasts. Friend cells cultured for 4 years are almost negative to conjugated antibody staining although they still preserve the erythrocyte expression, and could thus be considered from the viewpoint of erythrogenic expression as stem cells at the level of erythropoietin-reacting cells (ERc). In other words, the epigenotype of the Friend cells is already determined to be in the direction of the erythroid series. The differentiation of Friend cells is the release of the previously arrested maturation of these cells. Thus, the mechanism of leukemogenesis of Friend disease and differentiation of Friend cells seem to be very close.

2. MEM-antigens as a Marker of Erythroid Cells

In order to study the distribution of MEM-antigens, various kinds of cultured cells and transplantable tumor cells originating from the human, mouse, rat, and Chinese hamster were examined by conjugated antibody staining. Only 2 of 15 cell lines were positive to this staining. They were Friend cells of TSFAT-3-C1-1 and cultured erythroid cells (SLA cells) which originated from erythroleukemia cells of a female Sprague-Dawley rat induced by N-nitrosobutylurea. Therefore, the cell with MEM-antigens can be identified as an erythroid cell. The distribution of MEM-antigens in the Friend cells treated with effective substances was not limited to the cell surface. The antigens were also distributed diffusely in the cytoplasm and sometimes also in the perinuclear area. The ultrastructural location of the antigens was uncertain. According to preliminary results by electron microscopy, the polyribosome-rich areas in the cytoplasm may correspond to the fluorescence-positive regions. In the DMSO-treated cells, the virus-containing vacuoles in the cytoplasm may be closely related to the dots which are markedly positive to the fluorescent-antibodies. In the cells treated with N-dimethyl-rifampicin, the numerous submembranous fine dots could correspond to pinocytotic vesicles. The results may indicate a relationship between a newly formed cytoplasmic membrane and synthesis of MEM-antigens.

3. Virus Particles in the Treated Cells

In vivo experiments suggested a close relationship between virus particles and erythrocytic expression but this was not clear in *in vitro* experiments. Many virus particles were visible in the cytoplasmic vesicles of Friend cells treated with DMSO as they were in the cells in the *in vivo* experiments. Sato *et al.* [34] reported similar findings. The cells treated with N-dimethyl-rifampicin and Bleomycin gave a strong fluorescence and showed few virus particles in the cytoplasm. BudR markedly induced virus particles outside the cells, but the induction of MEM-antigens was not observed. Thus, there was no parallel relationship between activation of the viral genome and induction of antigens. MACPHERSON [25] reported that a revertant of kidney cells transformed by Rous sarcoma virus contained no viral genome, and POLLACK *et al.* [27] showed that a revertant of tumor cells induced by SV40 contained viral antigens. Therefore, although the possibility cannot be denied in special cases, the change of phenotypic expression or reversion may have no direct relation to the expression of the viral genome.

4. Groups of Substances Enhancing the MEM-antigens of Friend Cells

The *in vitro* experiments demonstrated that the induction or enhancement of MEM-antigens could occur under various conditions and with various substances. These conditions and substances will be divided into two groups; the inhibitors of DNA synthesis and the others. As indicated in Table 6, anticancer agents, and cultures kept at a low temperature or without serum belong like the inhibitors of DNA synthesis to the former group (Group 1), and Ep, VB_{12}, DMSO, N-dimethyl-rifampicin, rifamide, and glycerin, to the latter (Group 2). Except for cultures kept at low temperatures or without serum, the cells became larger by treatment with Group 1 substances and the induction of MEM-antigens was clearly demonstrable as early as the 2nd day. At the most effective dose cell growth was inhibited. The substances belonging to Group 1 are specific inhibitors of DNA synthesis and have drastic effects on the Friend cells. On the other hand, the cells treated with the Group 2 substances became smaller, induction of the antigens increased gradually, and became prominent on the 4th day. At the most effective dose the cells grew relatively well. These latter findings were similar to those found with cells cultured in diffusion chambers *in vivo*. With respect to these results, it should be said that the effect of the Group 2 compounds resembles the erythroid differentiation in normal hematopoiesis. Differentiation is observed not only in Friend cells but in some other tumor cells. Probably almost all tumor cells could be differentiated, the conditions

Table 6. Grouping of substances enhancing MEM-antigens

	Group 1	Group 2
Substance	Ara-C FudR Hydroxyurea	Combination of: Erythropoietin VB_{12} $(But)_2$-cAMP
	Bleomycin	DMSO
	MMC	N-dimethyl-rifampicin Cultured in diffusion chamber
Induction of antigens	early	late
Cell size	large	small
Growth	markedly inhibited	slightly inhibited

required to induce the differentiation varying for the different tumors. There is another cultured erythroid leukemia cell line (SLA-cells) in our laboratory. The SLA cells treated with the inhibitors of DNA synthesis showed a strong fluorescence in the cytoplasm when examined by the conjugated antibody technique.

Ep and VB_{12} were also effective for enhancement of MEM-antigens although DMSO was ineffective (our unpublished data). Therefore, there should be two different groups of substances which induce differentiation of tumor cells; one group including substances which are effective for many different tumors, and the other containing substances which show a specific effect on a particular tumor. The inhibitors of DNA synthesis are examples of the former and DMSO an example of the latter. Both groups are useful for obtaining information on the mechanism of differentiation of tumor cells. It is necessary to find a substance which is specifically effective for a given tumor.

An understanding of the mechanism of differentiation of a tumor might give us fundamental knowledge on the nature of cancer and on the control of cancer growth.

Conclusion

There is much evidence that the character of a tumor cell, i.e. the cancer phenotype, is not always stable but is able to change. Terms such as reversion, differentiation, and decarcinogenesis are used.

For example, that a long-term cultured Friend cell is able to differentiate along the erythrocytic series following treatment with some substances, can be demonstrated by the conjugated erythrocyte membrane-specific antibody technique. Differentiation may be induced by inhibition of DNA synthesis which is an artificial and drastic treatment, and by other more natural agents which are specific to Friend cells. Both ways are useful for obtaining information on the mechanism of differentiation of Friend cells. The expression of the viral genome incorporated into a cell seems not to be directly related to the differentiation of Friend cells. An understanding of the mechanism of differentiation of tumor cells may lead to a deeper insight into carcinogenesis, the nature of a tumor, and the control of tumor growth.

References

1. Adachi, H., Furusawa, M.: Exp. Cell Res. **50**, 490 (1968).
2. Biedler, J. L., Riehm, H.: Proc. Amer. Ass. Cancer Res. **11**, 30 (1970).
3. Blume, A., Gilbert, F., Wilson, S., Farber, J., Rosenberg, R., Nierenberg, M.: Proc. nat. Acad. Sci. (Wash.) **67**, 786 (1970).
4. Braun, A. C.: The cancer problem. New York, London: Columbia Univ. Press 1969.
5. Burger, M. M., Noonan, K. D.: Nature (Lond.) **228**, 512 (1970).
6. Everson, T. C., Cole, W. H.: Spontaneous regression of cancer. Philadelphia, London: W. B. Saunders 1966.
7. Friend, C.: J. exp. Med. **105**, 307 (1957).
8. Friend, C., Patuleia, M. C., de Harven, E.: Nat. Inst. Monogr. **22**, 505 (1966).
9. Friend, C., Scher, W., Holland, J. G., Sato, T.: Proc. nat. Acad. Sci. (Wash.) **68**, 378 (1971).
10. Furusawa, M., Adachi, H.: Exp. Cell. Res. **50**, 497 (1968).
11. Furusawa, M., Ikawa, Y., Sugano, H.: Proc. Jap. Acad. **47**, 220 (1971).
12. Furusawa, M., Takahashi, K. P.: Nature (Lond.) (in press) (1972).
13. Furusawa, M., Ikawa, Y., Sugano, H.: GANN Monogr. Cancer Res. **12**, 123 (1972).

14. GALLO, R. C., YANG, S. S., TING, R. C.: Nature (Lond.) **228**, 927 (1970).
15. GURGO, C., RAY, R. K., THIRY, L., GREEN, M.: Nature (Lond.) New Biol. **229**, 111 (1971)
16. HARRIS, H., MILLER, O. J., KLEIN, G., WORST, P., TACHIBANA, T.: Nature (Lond.) **223**, 363 (1969).
17. ICHIKAWA, Y.: J. cell. comp. Physiol. **76**, 175 (1970).
18. IKAWA, Y., SUGANO, H.: GANN **57**, 641 (1966).
19. IKAWA, Y., SUGANO, H.: Trans. Soc. path. Jap. **55**, 139 (1966).
20. IKAWA, Y., SUGANO, H., FURUSAWA, M.: GANN Monogr. Cancer Res. **12**, 29 (1972).
21. JOHNSON, G. S., FRIEDMAN, R. M., PASTON, I.: Proc. nat. Acad. Sci. (Wash.) **68**, 425 (1971).
22. KATES, J. R., WINTERTON, R., SCHLESSINGER, K.: Nature (Lond.) **229**, 345 (1971).
23. KASUGA, T.: Proc. Jap. Cancer Ass. (26th Ann. Meeting), p. 223 (1966).
24. KOYAMA, K., ISHII, K.: GANN **60**, 367 (1969).
25. MACPHERSON, I.: Science **148**, 1731 (1965).
26. PATULEIA, M. C., FRIEND, C.: Cancer Res. **27**, 726 (1967).
27. POLLACK, R., GREEN, H., TODARO, G.: Proc. nat. Acad. Sci. (Wash.) **60**, 126 (1968).
28. RABINOWITZ, A., SACHS, L.: Virology **40**, 193 (1970).
29. ROSSI, G. B., FRIEND, C.: Proc. nat. Acad. Sci. (Wash.) **58**, 1373 (1967).
30. ROTHCHILD, H., BLACK, P. H.: Proc. nat. Acad. Sci. (Wash.) **67**, 1042 (1970).
31. SANDERS, F. K., BURFORD, B. O.: Nature (Lond.) **220**, 448 (1968).
32. SASSA, S., TAKAKU, F., NAKAO, K., IKAWA, Y., SUGANO, H.: Proc. exp. biol. Med. **127**, 527 (1968).
33. SATO, S., MATSUSHIMA, T., SUGIMURA, T.: Cancer Res. **29**, 1437 (1969).
34. SATO, T., FRIEND, C., DE HARVEN, E.: Cancer Res. **31**, 1402 (1971).
35. SCHUBERT, D., JACOB, F.: Proc. nat. Acad. Sci. (Wash.) **67**, 247 (1970).
36. SILAGI, S., BRUCE, S. A.: Proc. nat. Acad. Sci. (Wash.) **66**, 72 (1970).
37. SOULE, H. D., ALBERT, S., WOLF, P. L., STANSLY, P. G.: Exp. Cell Res. **42**, 380 (1966).
38. SUGANO, H., FURUSAWA, M., KAWAGUCHI, T., IKAWA, Y.: 5th Intl. Symp. Comparative Leukemia Res., Padova (1971), Bibl. haemat. **39**, 943 (Karger: Basel 1973).
39. SUGANO, H., FURUSAWA, M., KAWAGUCHI, T., IKAWA, Y.: (in preparation).
40. SUGIMURA, T.: Chemical Tumor Problems. Ed. W. NAKAHARA. Tokyo: Jap. Soc. for the Promotion of Sci. 1970, pp. 269—284.
41. UMEZAWA, H., ISHIZUKA, M., KIMURA, K., IWANAGA, J., TAKEUCHI, T.: J. Antibiot. (Tokyo) **21**, 592 (1968).
42. UTAKOJI, T.: (personal communication).
43. YOSHIDA, T.: Meth. Cancer Res. **6**, 97 (1971).

Immunosuppressive Effect of Friend's Mouse Leukaemia and Anti-Thymocyte Serum on Herpes Simplex Virus Infection in Mice

K. MUNK and H. RUNNEBAUM

Clinical observations have revealed that infection with herpes viruses, such as herpes simplex virus, herpes zoster virus, varicella virus or cytomegalovirus can produce severe complications in patients at the terminal stage of neoplastic diseases, especially leukemias, or in those receiving immunosuppressive treatment following organ transplantation. From 611 reported clinical cases receiving organ transplants 125 developed complication from viral infections (MUNK and RUNNEBAUM, 1970). The majority of these complications were caused by herpes viruses. Because of these observations we investigated the immunosuppressive activity of Friend's mouse leukaemia virus (FLV) infection and antithymocyte serum (ATS) on herpes simplex virus (HSV) infection in mice. CEGLOWSKI and FRIEDMAN (1968 a, b, 1969, 1970) and FRIEDMAN and CEGLOWSKI (1968, 1971) conducted an extensive study of the immunosuppressive effect of FLV. These authors observed a reduction in antibody formation in FLV infected animals injected with sheep erythrocytes and E. coli, and concluded that FLV reduces the number of immuno competent lymphocytes. We developed this system further in order to analyze the mechanisms of reduced immune reaction to HSV infections. In addition, we applied ATS as another immunosuppressive factor. In the first series of experiments we investigated the reduction of resistance to HSV infection in mice previously infected with FLV. Resistance to infection was defined in terms of LD50 for mice receiving a standard HSV suspension. The results of these experiments showed that reduced resistance to HSV infection is an effect of previous FLV infection. A second series of experiments where ATS was applied as immunosuppressive agent also revealed a significant reduction in the resistance to HSV-infection in the ATS-treated mice.

Our results must be interpreted such that the cell-mediated immune reaction plays the dominant role in resistance to HSV infection and that this reaction is affected both by FLV infection and ATS-treatment. Thus we have demonstrated an experimental approach to the problem of the mechanisms of the immune reaction in neoplasias against viral infection. These approaches may be important for clinical considerations. The results from the reported cases where herpes virus infection predominantly cause complications in these patients suggest that one should pay more attention to latent virus infections of herpes viruses in patients and in donors of blood or organs.

References

1. CEGLOWSKI, W. S., FRIEDMAN, H.: Proc. Soc. exp. Biol. (N. Y.) **126,** 662 (1968 a).
2. CEGLOWSKI, W. S., FRIEDMAN, H.: J. Immunol. **101,** 594 (1968 b).
3. CEGLOWSKI, W. S., FRIEDMAN, H.: J. Immunol. **102,** 338 (1969).
4. CEGLOWSKI, W. S., FRIEDMAN, H.: J. Immunol. **105,** 1406 (1970).
5. FRIEDMAN, H., CEGLOWSKI, W. S.: Nature (Lond.) **218,** 1232 (1968).
6. FRIEDMAN, H., CEGLOWSKI, W. S.: J. Immunol. **107,** 1673 (1971).
7. MUNK, K., RUNNEBAUM, H.: Dtsch. med. Wschr. **95,** 2252 (1970).

Precancerous Lesions and their Detection and Diagnosis

L. G. Koss

This meeting marks almost to the day the 21st anniversary of my involvement in cytology. When as a young pathologist I first decided to explore this field, the views of my then superiors and contemporaries were decidedly negative.

Nevertheless I moved on to the Memorial Hospital where I met Dr. PAPANICOLAOU, who was then consultant in cytology. He used to come twice a week to the dark and uncomfortable little laboratory in the basement of the Strang Cancer Prevention Clinic building and review some of the more interesting cases. PAPANICOLAOU was an anatomist who knew little pathology and lived in mortal fear of a diagnostic mistake. He was therefore very cautious and, rather than commit himself to a definitive diagnosis, elected to render his opinions as "classes" of smears. He rarely committed himself to a classification higher than Class IV (presumable cancer), unless the evidence was absolutely overwhelming. His favored diagnosis on abnormal smears was "Class III" or suspicious; that he soon subdivided into Class III A and III B, to indicate a lesser or greater degree of suspicion.

PAPANICOLAOU made many basic contributions to the recognition of carcinoma in situ and related lesions of the uterine cervix and other organs. He observed that cells from the earliest precancerous lesions of cervix epithelium are quite different from cells of carcinoma in situ and from cells of invasive carcinoma. To describe the cells from the earliest lesions he coined the term "dyskaryosis" to define cells with a cancerous nucleus and a nearly normal cytoplasm.

He also made many basic contributions to the cytology of other organs. His Atlas [18] is a remarkable compendium of cells and cell types, a massive accumulation of experience, not always well correlated with histologic findings, but forever a monument to the power of perception and observation of GEORGE NICHOLAS PAPANICOLAOU.

The Uterine Cervix

It is perhaps of interest to note that PAPANICOLAOU cannot claim priority to the most widely used application of cytology, detection of cancer of the uterine cervix. The credit here goes to a Roumanian pathologist, AURELI BABES who, some months before PAPANICOLAOU, published an article on diagnosis of cancer of the cervix by smears [1]. Whether the credit goes to PAPANICOLAOU or to BABES is immaterial in view of the successful application of cytology to the detection of precancerous states of the cervix. Carcinoma in situ of the cervix prior to 1950 was a rarity observed only in a few specialized institutions either as a result of colposcopy or of a chance biopsy; now it is a common pathologic entity. In fact, to many of the younger generation of pathologists in the United States invasive cancer of the cervix has become a rarity, whereas they may observe carcinoma in situ on a daily basis.

No significant doubt remains in the minds of serious observers of carcinoma in situ that the lesion, if untreated, will progress in many but not all cases to invasive carcinoma of cervix. For instance, KOTTMEIER observed 34 patients with this disease without treatment; 25 of them developed invasive cervix cancer within a follow-up period of 2 to 21 years [13].

The question still unresolved in the minds of many is that of definitions. About 10 years ago, an international committee of experts arbitrarily defined carcinoma *in situ* of the cervix as a lesion without surface differentiation. Nothing could be further from the truth, as any working pathologist will attest. Carcinoma *in situ* of the cervix is by definition a lesion that looks like cancer and hence is capable of differentiation and keratin formation [6]. In its most recent deliberations the WHO committee on uterine tumors fortunately recognized this fact and soon hopefully the old definition will be permanently discarded.

Another, more significant problem pertains to the lesions of lesser degree of abnormality that cannot qualify as carcinomas in situ. These lesions are characterized better by their cytologic abnormalities than by the histologic patterns; the latter may be inconspicuous and require a practiced eye for recognition.

These lesions have received various names from "atypisches Epithel" to anaplasia, dysplasia or borderline lesions. For a long time all major significance was denied to these lesions. Careful studies disclosed, however, that such lesions are in equal measure precursors of invasive cancer of the cervix as the more classical carcinoma *in situ* [7, 12].

Our own investigation [12] conducted for over 10 years in New York City, disclosed several important facts about carcinoma *in situ* and borderline lesions (mild and moderate dysplasia), some of which may be summarized as follows:

1. A simple punch biopsy may significantly alter the distribution and natural history of these lesions. As a consequence, post-biopsy studies of these lesions do not reflect their true behavior.

2. Histologic or cytologic patterns do not lend themselves to prognostication. Any epithelial lesion with nuclear abnormalities may lead to carcinoma *in situ* or to invasive carcinoma of the cervix.

3. If followed under uniform conditions of observation, carcinoma *in situ* and dysplasia show strikingly similar behavior patterns with an approximately equal percentage of lesions disappearing after biopsy. The progression of mild and moderate dysplasia to carcinoma *in situ* occurred in 40% of cases.

Similar conclusions pertaining to dysplasia as a progressive lesion were reached by RICHART and BARRON [20]. STERN and NEELY [27] pointed out that women with dysplasia have a 1,600 times greater chance of developing carcinoma *in situ* than women without this disease. It has also been documented that dysplasias have an abnormal chromosomal makeup, akin to that of invasive carcinoma [26].

4. Perhaps the most important lesson from the study of carcinoma *in situ* and related lesions of the uterine cervix pertains to the natural history of precancerous states and cancer in man. It has been clearly shown that cancer is not the acute disease that it once was thought to be. On the contrary, the slow and unpredictable progression of the precancerous epithelial lesions that may last as long as 20 years

and may never result in clinical cancer appears to be the rule rather than the exception. In a recent publication [7] I compared cancer of the uterine cervix to an iceberg: only a small portion of it is visible on the surface in the form of clinical disease; most of its natural history is spent in preparation for the final events.

If the usage of cytology in the detection and diagnosis of precancerous lesions of the cervix has received wide popular support, the same does not apply to other organs. Yet, sophisticated observers may achieve diagnostic results that closely match those recorded for the uterine cervix.

The Endometrium

Cytologic diagnosis of precancerous states and early carcinoma of the endometrium is entirely possible, provided that an adequate source of cells is available. A cervical smear is obviously not suited for this purpose. Our own successes were based on the examination of a vaginal pool smear [9]. REAGAN and NG [19] achieved good results with endocervical aspirations. In my opinion, the simplest and most effective method of endometrial cancer detection remains the vaginal pool smear. This should be routinely obtained on every woman past 40 years of age.

Cytologic detection programs of endometrial carcinoma focused our attention on a number of interesting problems. The asymptomatic patient was often still menstruating regularly when the lesion was discovered. Nearly all patients with early lesions detected by cytology showed an excellent maturation of vaginal squamous epithelium reflecting hormonal activity — much in contrast with women with advanced endometrial carcinoma, about half of whom had no evidence of residual hormonal effect. BERG and DURFEE, working in my laboratory, calculated that women with good hormonal effect past their clinical menopause had a 15 times greater chance of developing carcinoma of the endometrium than women with pattern of postmenopausal atrophy [2].

Another interesting observation pertained to histiocytes or histiocytic-like cells that accompany endometrial cancer cells. Somewhat similar cells may be observed at the end of the normal menstrual bleeding; they appear to originate from endometrial stromal cells. The histiocytic transformation of endometrial stroma may be observed in cancer as well. Occasionally the presence of such cells in vaginal smears may herald endometrial carcinoma [6].

If one recognizes the form of endometrial cancer named by HERTIG *et al.* [5] carcinoma *in situ*, several such lesions were identified cytologically in both asymptomatic and symptomatic patients. It is of interest that the average age of a group of 13 patients with this lesion was 52 whereas the average age for fully developed carcinoma of endometrium was 57 years of age. This would suggest that 5 years are required for progression of carcinoma *in situ* to invasive cancer — a figure well in keeping with our current knowledge of natural history of human cancer [6].

The Urinary Bladder

The urinary bladder is another primary target organ for cytologic diagnosis of cancer. We are particularly concerned here with sessile non-papillary carcinoma *in situ*, a form of bladder cancer that only recently received full recognition as a result of cytologic screening and follow-up studies of industrial workers exposed to potent bladder carcinogens [10, 11].

Of particular interest to us is non-papillary carcinoma *in situ* as a primary lesion. In common with other carcinomas *in situ* the lesion produces no specific signs or symptoms [16]. Clinically there is evidence of nonspecific cystitis, occasionally with microscopic hematuria. Cytoscopically the lesions masquerade as areas of redness or inflammation. Cytology of the urinary sediment discloses cancer cells of a rather peculiar, round, uniform appearance [6]. This is in contrast to cytologic findings in fully invasive carcinoma where the variability of cancer cells is quite striking.

There is good evidence that the majority if not all carcinomas *in situ* of the bladder will progress to invasive cancer capable of metastases within a few years. There are not enough cases carefully followed and reported to obtain statistically valid information on the average duration of this process. However, invasive carcinoma of bladder was observed in 11 out of 13 industrial workers with carcinoma *in situ* [10]. Utz *et al.* [28] recorded 80% recurrence in 62 patients with this disease and Yates Bell [29] recently published 4 cases, all leading to invasive carcinoma.

Similarly, sessile carcinoma *in situ* of the bladder occurring after prior treatment of papillary tumors also has a grave prognosis. In Melamed's series of 19 cases, invasive carcinoma occurred in 8 cases after a follow-up period ranging from 10 to 68 months [16]. Schade and Swinney [25] demonstrated carcinoma *in situ* and other significant abnormalities adjacent to invasive carcinoma in 80% of cases.

There is little doubt that the sessile, non-papillary carcinoma *in situ* as the initial lesion of bladder cancer is less frequent than other proliferative processes such as papilloma, papillary carcinoma or hyperplasia. It is therefore possible that 2 distinct processes of cancerogenesis occur in human urinary bladder: the rather slowly progressing proliferative epithelial disease, manifested by hyperplasia, papillomas and papillary carcinomas and the more rapidly progressing non-papillary cancer with carcinoma *in situ* as its first manifestation.

The Lung

Competently performed cytologic examination of sputum is an indispensable part of a careful examination of any patient with chronic cough or with roentgenologic evidence of pulmonary abnormalities. Eighty percent of lung cancers can be accurately diagnosed in this fashion. The remainder, usually peripherally located lesions, are accessible to other forms of cytologic diagnosis, either by intrabronchial brush method [4] or by aspiration biopsy [3].

Perhaps the most important contribution of sputum cytology to the solution of the problem of lung cancer is the diagnosis of bronchogenic carcinoma *in situ* or at a very early invasive stage where cure by surgical resection is possible [15]. Such cases often fail to show any roentgenologic manifestations of disease. The clinical symptomatology is usually persisting cough, usually productive of sputum and occasionally with evidence of hemoptysis. A painstaking cytologic examination of sputum is necessary in such cases.

Nasiell [17] and Saccomanno *et al.* [21] pointed out that cytologic changes reflecting atypical squamous metaplasia of bronchial epithelium, often preceding bronchogenic carcinoma, may be observed in sputum. Saccomanno *et al.* [22] pointed out that occasionally such cytologic findings may be used in prognosticating the outcome of the metaplastic changes. Should this observation be confirmed, cytology of sputum will become an indispensable tool in the follow-up of patients with chronic cough or other symptoms referable to bronchial disease, particularly if such patients have been exposed to known carcinogenic agents such as uranium or asbestos.

Buccal Cavity and Gastrointestinal Tract

Similar successes have been recorded with cancer of the buccal cavity and the upper gastrointestinal tract, mainly the esophagus and the stomach. Studies of SANDLER [23] demonstrated clearly that carcinoma in situ of the buccal cavity is usually not recognized as such. Again, these early forms of cancer masquerade as areas of redness or inflammation. Cytologic examination of scrapings of all lesions of buccal cavity contributed substantially to the identification of carcinoma in situ exept in situations where the lesions were heavily keratinized.

There are on record several cases of esophageal carcinoma *in situ* diagnosed by cytology. However, there is no sustained study of this lesion [6].

Gastric carcinoma *in situ* on the other hand has been extensively studied by SCHADE in England [24] and by the Japanese workers [14]. The target of SCHADE's studies were patients with chronic gastritis and pernicious anemia. The Japanese workers adressed themselves to large groups of populations, combining cytology with fibergastroscopies and gastric cameras with remarkable results.

Summary

This brief summary of accomplishments of cytology within the realm of early cancer detection does not by any means exhaust the possibilities of this technique. Numerous clinical situations lend themselves to evaluation by cytology, be it by examination of various body fluids, be it by aspiration of various organs.

As a pathologist, I must stress the great need for constant correlation of cytologic findings with histologic observations and the need for a careful clinical follow-up. Diagnostic cytology, like any other form of morphologic diagnosis, does not belong in the hands of amateurs but rather must be practiced by carefully trained professionals. Only then will the benefits of this method of diagnosis become universal.

References

1. BABES, A.: Presse méd. **36**, 451 (1928).
2. BERG, J. W., DURFEE, G. R.: Cancer (Philad.) **11**, 158 (1958).
3. DAHLGREN, S., NORDENSTRÖM, B.: Transthoracic needle biopsy, Stockholm, Sweden: Almqvist & Wiksells 1966.
4. HATTORI, S., MATSUDA, M., SUGIYAMA, T., MATSUDA, H.: Dis. Chest **45**, 129 (1964).
5. HERTIG, A. T., SOMMERS, S. C., BENGLOFF, H.: Cancer (Philad.) **2**, 964 (1949).
6. KOSS, L. G.: Diagnostic cytology and its histopathologic bases. 2nd ed. Philadelphia: Lippincott 1968.
7. KOSS, L. G.: Obstet. gynec. Surv. **24**, 850 (1969).
8. KOSS, L. G.: Clin. Obstet. Gynec. **13**, 873 (1970).
9. KOSS, L. G., DURFEE, G. R.: Acta cytol. (Philad.) **6**, 519 (1962).
10. KOSS, L. G., MELAMED, M. R., KELLY, R. E.: J. nat. Cancer Inst. **43**, 233 (1969).

11. Koss, L. G., Melamed, M. R., Ricci, A., Melick, W. F., Kelly, R. E.: New Engl. J. Med. **272**, 676 (1965).
12. Koss, L. G., Stewart, F. W., Foote, F. W., Jordan, M. J., Bader, G. M., Day, E.: Cancer (Philad.) **16**, 1160 (1963).
13. Kottmeier, H. L.: Personal communication dated Aug. 2, 1968 quoted in Reference 7.
14. Kurokawa, T., Kajitani, T., Oota, K.: Carcinoma of the stomach in early phase. Tokyo: Nakayama-Shoten Co., Ltd. 1967.
15. Melamed, M. R., Koss, L. G., Cliffton, E. E.: Cancer (Philad.) **16**, 1537 (1963).
16. Melamed, M. R., Voutsa, N. G., Grabstald, H.: Cancer (Philad.) **17**, 1533 (1964).
17. Nasiell, M.: The epithelial picture in the bronchial mucosa in chronic inflammatory and neoplastic lung disease and its relation to smoking. A comparative histologic and sputum-cytologic study. Stockholm: Tryckeribolaget Ivar Haggström AB 1968.
18. Papanicolaou, G. N.: Atlas of exfoliative cytology. Commonwealth Fund by Harvard University Press, Cambridge, Mass. 1963.
19. Reagan, J. W., Ng, A. B. P.: The cells of uterine adenocarcinoma. Monograph. Basel (Switzerland): Karger; Baltimore: Williams & Wilkins 1965.
20. Richart, R. M., Barron, B. A.: Amer. J. Obstet. Gynec. **105**, 386 (1969).
21. Saccomanno, G., Saunders, R. P., Archer, V. E., Aerbach, O., Kuschner, M., Beckler, P.: Acta cytol. (Philad.) **9**, 413 (1965).
22. Saccomanno, G., Saunders, R. P., Klein, M. G., Archer, V. E., Brennan, L.: Acta cytol. (Philad.) **14**, 377 (1970).
23. Sandler, H. C.: Cancer (Philad.) **15**, 1119 (1962).
24. Schade, R. O. K.: Acta cytol. (Philad.) **3**, 7 (1959).
25. Schade, R. O. K., Swinney, J.: Lancet **1968 II**, p. 943.
26. Spriggs, A. I., Bowey, C. E., Cowdell, R. H.: Cancer (Philad.) **27**, 1239 (1971).
27. Stern, E., Neely, P. M.: Cancer (Philad.) **17**, 508 (1964).
28. Utz, D. C., Hanash, K. A., Farrow, G. M.: J. Urol. (Baltimore) **103**, 160 (1970).
29. Yates-Bell, A. J.: Brit. J. Surg. **58**, 359 (1971).

Preinvasive Carcinoma

H. Hamperl

The term "preinvasive cancer", or its more common synonym "carcinoma *in situ*", is nowadays being freely applied to an ever increasing number of lesions in different organs. The terms are used to describe not only a special form of the growth of a cancer, but also a stage in cancer development which implies that sooner or later the cancer will shift into the typical invasive growth form. In this latter sense they become wideley known and accepted.

The term "pre-invasive cancer" in this sense has been applied to lesions of the cervix uteri, which has proved to be an ideal location for the study of the possible changes in the epithelial covering by use of such methods as colposcopy, cytology, histochemistry and cytophotometry. At other sites, such as in the mammary gland where "lobular carcinomas *in situ*" have been described, the application of these methods is not always so easy. Even more difficult has been the task of detecting and following the development and growth of what is now called "cancer *in situ*" of the mucous membranes of the stomach or intestine.

Without doubt all the lesions described, and also some lesions long known under other names, but now incorporated under the heading "carcinoma in situ" (e. g. Bowens disease of the skin, keratosis senilis and erythroplasia) show common traits, but they also show some differences. Consequently although in discussing the significance of carcinoma *in situ* we shall refer primarily to carcinoma *in situ* of the cervix uteri, we should not forget that other types of carcinoma *in situ* can also provide important information.

The question around which discussing is centered is the following: is a carcinoma *in situ* already a carcinoma or only a stage in the development of a carcinoma? The answer holds important consequences for the diagnosis, treatment and prevention of the cancers of different organs. The carcinoma *in situ* of the cervix and, to a certain degree, the lobular cancer *in situ* of the breast were first treated with the *radical measures* commonly applied to the invasive carcinomas and therapy was reported as being almost 100% successful. In addition cases were recorded in which an excision from the cervix or the breast was made, the diagnosis established, but the patient subsequently not treated for one reason or another. Surprisingly nothing happened in many untreated patients; they developped neither recurrencies nor metastases. Several explanations have been offered to explain these unexpected observations.

1. It was suggested that the carcinoma had been *entirely removed* by the excision. However, it was pointed out that in some cases portions of the carcinoma *in situ* must have been left behind, since the line of excision passed through the lesion.

2. It was proposed that a tumor in the stage of carcinoma *in situ* is *especially vulnerable*, so that local inflammation developing after excision was sufficient to destroy the remaining tumor cells.

3. Finally, the suspicion arose, that the *diagnosis* of the lesion was *not correct*. It is in fact very difficult to establish exact boundary lines between dysplasia and carcinoma *in situ*. When diagnoses submitted by different pathologists for the same lesion of the cervix were compared, the results were rather discouraging as they often differed greatly. In the breast the uncertainty of the histological diagnosis of the lobular carcinoma *in situ* was at least as great. The reason for this is that there are not only several types of carcinoma lobulare *in situ* each possibly behaving differently, but also several lesions mimicking the carcinoma *in situ* to such an extent, that McDIVITT *et al.* (1968) found it necessary to devote a major part of the fascicle on mammary tumors in the tumor atlas to just this differential diagnosis.

When we summarize these facts we are left *uncertain* as to whether the carcinoma *in situ* is really the smallest carcinoma still confined to the site of its origin or rather a lesion belonging to a kind of precursor state.

There exists a tendency to solve the dilemma by simply stating that the lesion we call carcinoma *in situ* is *histologically malignant* and can be called "cancer" by the pathologist, but on the other hand that it is *clinically benign*. Here we find ourselves on very dangerous ground. One could and should consequently ask: who should decide wether or not a given tumor is malignant — the histologist or the clinician? Although I am a pathologist I have to admit, that the notion of malignancy stemmed from clinical observation whereas the histopathological observation and classification came only in its wake. The statement "clinically benign, histologically malignant" can, therefore, not be accepted as making any sense. If a certain lesion is found by careful clinical observation to be behave like a benign one, then no histological analogy or similarity with a malignant lesion can alter the conclusions drawn from the clinical observation. It is up the pathologist to mend his ways and conform to the clinical realities. Simply to classify, as some do, a certain lesion as a benign carcinoma, is an inadmissible "contradictio in adjecto", like speaking of a white negro. If we admit that benign carcinomas exist we *deprive the term carcinoma of all significance and usefulness* in the communication between clinician and pathologist. Patients untainted by medical or pathological knowledge react to the term "carcinoma *in situ*" in a quite natural way: they hear the word "carcinoma" and invariably associate it with malignancy and all its direct consequences. It is a difficult task to explain to them how the additional words "*in situ*" deprive the term "carcinoma" of just what it is generally meant to signify. Unfortunately these misunderstandings are not confined to lay people but are shared by some physicians, resulting in unnecessary radical therapy. We are, therefore, frequently asked: "Why does one call lesion a 'carcinoma' when one is convinced that it will not behave as one is accustomed to believe carcinomas should behave?"

17 years ago German pathologists and clinicians (HAMPERL and KAUFMANN, 1956) felt this question weighing heavily on their consciences and tentatively recommended the use of a nomenclature originally proposed by HINSELMANN. He recognized the lesion we now call carcinoma *in situ* of the cervix only as "*highly atypical epithelium*". In the long run, however, the import from the USA outweighed the export from Germany and we were obliged to adopt the term carcinoma *in situ* in the sense now

used in the USA. It was too late to change the use of a term so generally accepted there to signify a definite histological picture. In a similar way a precancerous lesion of the breast (McDIVITT *et al.*, 1967) presently known as a carcinoma lobulare *in situ* was called a "*solid intracanalicular outgrowth of epithelia*" by BÖHMIG (1952). Today the term "carcinoma lobulare *in situ*" is considered "most unfortunate" by HAAGENSEN (1971), who would like to replace it by "lobular neoplasia" for the reasons previously discussed.

The patho-histological analogies and similarities between a carcinoma *in situ* and a typical malignant tumor cannot, therefore, be accepted as convincing evidence of its malignancy as long it is not corroborated by clinical behaviour. Without any doubt the histological picture of a carcinoma *in situ* of the cervix very closely resembles that of typical carcinomas, showing cellular polymorphism, frequent mitoses, atypical mitoses, the loss of regular cellular arrangement and stratification, as well as other identical characteristics detected histochemically and cytologically. All these common factors should not, however, obscure other differences between a typical carcinoma and the carcinoma *in situ*. According to our present knowledge a carcinoma is thought to originate from a definite group of cells. It has been experimentally possible to transplant a malignant tumor by the transfer of a single cell. The progeny of that cell, or cells, multiply unchecked by the normal regulatory mechanisms.

During the last few years detailed observations have indicated that the carcinoma *in situ* may originate and grow in another way: As JOHNSON *et al.* (1964) and BURGHARDT (1972) have shown, the carcinoma *in situ* of the cervix begins with atypical growth of all the basal cells in a certain area. With time the abnormal cells replace the whole thickness of the stratified epithelium from the base to the surface. Such areas may remain and border immediately on normal cells. If such an area expands it does not replace the normal cells by infiltrating or pushing them aside, but by inducing the adjacent normal basal cells to join them in their abnormal growth. We observed essentially similar behaviour in the lobular carcinoma *in situ* of the breast (HAMPERL, 1972). From a purely morphological point of view one would call this kind of growth a "*growth by apposition*", which is alien to true carcinomas. How this spreading induction works remains obscure: but it is possible that the same stimulus which provoked the abnormal growth in the first area is then acting on a new area, or that an atypically growing cell induces the change in a neighbouring cell. This is what SPEEMANN (1926) called "induction".

Finally, the fact which sets the carcinoma *in situ* apart from the malignant tumor is that the *onset* of *invasion* is an event which *fundamentally changes the whole character of the lesion* and its finer morphology. Paradoxically the invading cancerous epithelia in the cervix may lose the polymorphy of the *in situ*-phase and even show signs of differentiation. In the mammary gland the invading cancer cells assume the appearance of a scirrhous carcinoma with ample production of connective tissue and even small intracellular cavities lined by microvilli.

The fundamental step required to transform a carcinoma *in situ* to an invasive carcinoma relegates the carcinoma *in situ* to the position of a qualitatively different lesion, or in other words to a precursor of cancer, a precancer.

Actually the term carcinoma *in situ* is being increasingly used in this sense. The situation becomes clearer if one includes, as is now generally done, Bowen's disease, keratosis senilis and erythroplasia in the category of carcinoma *in situ*. Dermatologists long ago considered these lesions to be potential cancers, but would undoubtedly object strongly if one called them cancers in the sense of an actually malignant invasive tumor.

Summary

The term "carcinoma *in situ*" in the meaning of precancer has been indiscriminately applied to many lesions in various organs (for exemple uterine cervix, stomach, intestine, prostate, urinary bladder and many others). It is too late to stop this trend, but not too late to point out the dangerous blurring of the boundaries between the terms cancer, meaning a clinically malignant growth, and carcinoma *in situ* meaning a pre-cancerous lesion.

References

BÖHMIG, R.: Zbl. allg. Path. path. Anat. **89**, 297 (1952).
BURGHARDT, E.: Histologische Frühdiagnose des Zervixkrebses. Stuttgart: Thieme 1972.
HAAGENSEN, C. D.: Diseases of the Breast. Second Edition. Philadelphia, London, Toronto: W. B. Saunders Company 1971.
HAMPERL, H.: Z. Krebsforsch. **77**, 231 (1972).
HAMPERL, H., KAUFMANN, C.: Z. Krebsforsch. **61**, 255 (1956).
JOHNSON, L. D., EASTERDAY, C. L., GORE, H., HERTIG, A. T.: Cancer (Philad.) **17**, 213 (1964).
MCDIVITT, R. W., HUTTER, R. V. P., FOOTE, JR., F. W., STEWART, F. W.: J. Amer. med. Ass. **201**, 82 (1967).
MCDIVITT, R. W., STEWART, F. W., BERG, J. W.: Tumors of the Breast. Atlas of Tumor Pathology. 2nd Series. Fasc. 2. Armed Forces Institute of Pathology, Washington D. C. 1968.
SPEEMANN, H.: Experimentelle Beiträge zu einer Theorie der Entwicklung. Berlin: Springer 1926.

Enzyme Histochemistry of Human Tumors

Indications of Differentiation and Functioning

R. G. J. Willighagen and A. C. Nieuwenhuyzen-Kruseman

The value of histochemical enzyme reactions in the study of human tumors for clinical-pathological purposes has been extensively investigated in many laboratories. Such studies have also been made in our department during the past 18 years (Willighagen 1956, 1959, 1960, 1961 a, b, 1963; Willighagen *et al.* 1959, 1963, 1968; Planteydt *et al.* 1960, 1965; Thiery *et al.* 1966, 1967 a, b, 1969).

Another aspect of studies of enzyme histochemistry in human and experimental tumors is the relationship between enzyme activity and tumor-cell differentiation: this differentiation can be morphological and/or functional. Morphological differentiation can be observed in all tumors as a degree of specialization, for example, cornification in squamous-cell carcinomas, adenostructures with secretion in adenocarcinomas, collagen formation in fibromas and fibrosarcomas. These phenomena are also expressions of functional differentiation. Other examples of functional differentiation can be found in tumors of endocrine organs which are able to produce hormones.

The morphological differentiation, the functioning of tumor cells, and the activity of enzymes are expressions of genetic information, present in all cells, and which can also be present in tumor cells. In many human tumors the histochemically demonstrable activity of enzymes is correlated with morphological differentiation and hormone production.

This is, however, not necessarily so. One might expect that, when the process of differentiation or functioning of the tumor cell is dependent on one or more enzymes, these enzymes should be demonstrable in the differentiated tumor cell. Much of the histochemically demonstrable enzyme activity in normal and tumor cells, however, is not clearly related to the process of differentiation. Such enzymes can be depleted in tumor cells without influencing the process of differentiation. It is therefore remarkable that in many differentiated tumor cells these enzymes are still present, although not always. Conversely, in undifferentiated tumors, the enzymes characteristic of the differentiated tumor cell may still be present. The association of histochemically demonstrable enzyme activity and morphological and functional differentiation can be demonstrated in many tumors.

Our first example illustrates the relationship between the activity of non-specific esterases and differentiation of squamous-cell carcinomas of the lung. In normal squamous epithelium a high activity of non-specific esterase can be demonstrated in the stratum granulosum. In lung tumors with cornification some activity of this enzyme is also seen in most cases. However, in squamous-cell carcinomas of the lung in which no cornification is present, activity of non-specific esterases may also be demonstrated in many tumors. The activity of esterases may be related in some unknown way with the process of keratinization; there is, however, no direct evidence of this. The relationship between the activity of esterases and keratinization is stressed by the investigation of YOSHIMURA *et al.* (1970), who demonstrated the presence of an isoenzyme of esterases in induced squamous-cell carcinomas and in normal skin. Squamous-cell carcinomas of the lung show that morphological differentiation is not always in parallel with the activity of an enzyme characteristic of the normal squamous epithelium.

We considered the possibility that the activity of the non-specific esterases in squamous-cell carcinomas of the lung without keratinization could be a more sensitive indication of differentiation in this group of tumors. Since in squamous-cell carcinomas of the lung a relationship exists between the degree of differentiation and the prognosis, we thought it sensible to start a follow-up study of the patients in whose surgical specimens we had studied the activity of esterases. We did this in order to establish whether there is a relationship between the activity of esterases and the biological behavior of these tumors. Fig. 1 shows the results of these studies. It is clear from these findings that there is a distinct correlation between the activity of esterases in squamous-cell carcinomas of the lung and the biological behavior of these tumors as expressed in survival time after operation. The activity of esterases is, in our opinion, a better indication than the morphological features for the grade of differentiation of the tumor cells.

Another example of deviation between morphological and enzymatic differentiation can be found in adenocarcinoma of the endometrium. In patients with adenocarcinoma of the endometrium treated with progesterone derivatives, we observed morphological and histochemical changes characteristic of secretion in the normal endometrium. The histochemical changes started earlier than the morphological

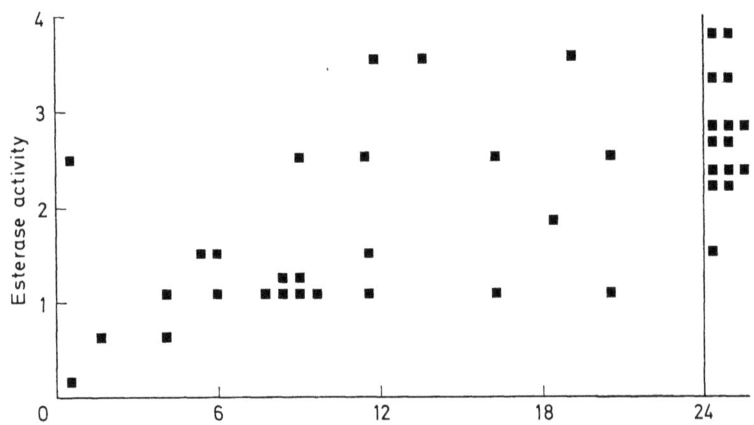

Fig. 1. Relative esterase activity and survival time of patients with squamous-cell carcinoma of the lung. Solid squares: deaths. Open squares: surviving patients

changes, which could not always be established. However, in one patient only morphological and no distinct histochemical changes were seen.

Fig. 2 shows how the activity of alkaline phosphatase in these patients changes after treatment with progesterone derivatives. Decreased enzyme activity was observed after prolonged treatment. This phenomenon was interpreted as secretory exhaustion, since the treatment can induce secretion in adenocarcinomas of the endometrium. Independent of the morphological differentiation by this treatment, changes can also be seen in the activity of enzymes that undergo cyclic changes in the normal endometrium.

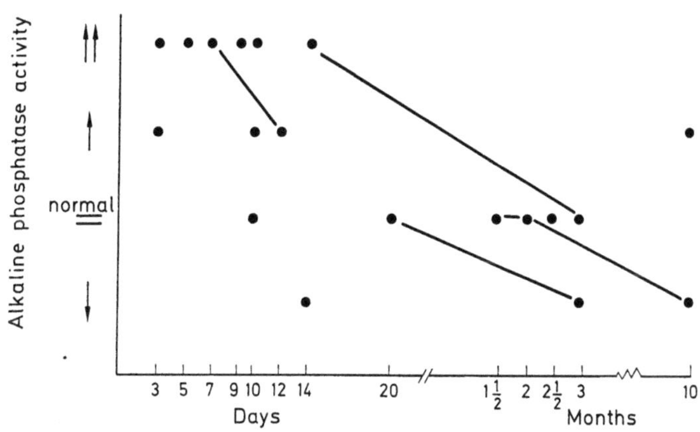

Fig. 2. Alkaline phosphatase activity in patients with adenocarcinoma of the endometrium before and after treatment with progesterone derivatives. Connecting lines indicate more than one biopsy in the same patient

Carcinomas of the adrenal cortex can produce different syndromes. Of the 18 carcinomas of the adrenal cortex we studied, 9 produced hormones. Five patients suffered from Cushing's syndrome, two had hyperaldosteronism and two had an oestrogen-producing tumor.

In both normal and experimental circumstances there is a relationship between the activity of glucose-6-phosphate dehydrogenase and 3-beta-ol-steroid dehydrogenase and hormone production. An enzyme characteristic of the adrenal cortex and many carcinomas of the adrenal cortex is alkaline phosphatase (VAN DE WEG, 1971). This last enzyme, however, is not related to hormone production. It is to be expected that the first two enzymes will be present in hormone-producing carcinomas, whereas the activity of alkaline phosphatase in carcinomas of the adrenal cortex can appear in the tumor cells independent of hormone production. On the other hand, the presence of glucose-6-phosphate dehydrogenase does not necessarily indicate that an adrenal cortex carcinoma produces hormone. This enzyme acts as a NADP reductase to provide NADPH for hydroxylating processes during hormone synthesis. In our opinion, this part of the biochemical reaction can be present without complete hormone synthesis.

Table 1 presents the results of biochemical estimations for two adrenal cortex carcinomas, compared with the normal zona fasciculata of human adrenals. From

Table 1. Activity of enzymes in the adrenal cortex

Activity expressed in moles/kg dry tissue/h.	alkaline phosphatase	glucose-6-phosphate dehydrogenase	3-beta-ol-steroid dehydrogenase
Functioning tumor (Cushing)	0.3	7.5	7.0
Non-functioning tumor	0.2	2.7	0.0
Normal zone fasciculata	1.5—3.5	2.7—5.3	52—101

table 1 it can be seen that in this case the tumor glucose-6-phosphate dehydrogenase activity is higher than that of the normal cortex. The activity of 3-beta-ol-steroid dehydrogenase in this hormone-producing tumor is much lower than in the normal adrenal cortex. The total mass of the tumor, however, accounted for the increased steroid production in this patient.

It was demonstrated in this group that enzymes necessary for hormone production are always present in hormone-producing tumors of the adrenal cortex, whereas in non-functioning tumors these enzymes may or may not be present. Alkaline phosphatase is present in normal adrenal cortex but is not related to hormone production. In 6 out of 9 non-functioning adrenal carcinomas this enzyme was absent; it was absent in only 2 out of 9 functioning carcinomas. There seems to be a correlation between the functional differentiation of these carcinomas and the activity of alkaline phosphatase, but it is not absolute.

Our last example concerns the activity of enzymes and functional differentiation as demonstrated in human lung carcinomas which produce ACTH. The material we studied histochemically included three lung tumors with a clinical syndrome of ACTH production. From the literature there is circumstantial evidence that these tumors are derived from the so-called APUD system (Pearse, 1968). This system was described in 1953 by Feyrter. Tumors of this system include, among others medullary carcinomas of the thyroid, carcinoids and insulomas.

We considered these facts together: ACTH-producing tumors are derived from APUD cells; carcinoids of the lung are also derived from APUD cells; there is a possibility that oat-cell carcinomas are undifferentiated carcinoids. As a result, we thought that lung tumors might produce ACTH in small amounts, without the clinical symptoms of Cushing's disease.

Therefore a combined study of ACTH immunofluorescence and enzyme histochemistry was started on a new series of lung tumors. The ACTH antibody was produced by immunization of rabbits with bovine ACTH. The APUD properties studied were the activities of non-specific esterases and mitochondrial alpha-glycerophosphate dehydrogenase. To our surprise, 7 out of 50 lung carcinomas showed presence of ACTH with the immunofluorescence method. In these tumors the activity of non-specific esterases was higher than in most other lung tumors; only in the squamous-cell carcinomas was the activity in the same range. The activity of mitochondrial alpha-glycerophosphate dehydrogenase was higher in most of the tumors with positive ACTH fluorescence than in those with negative fluorescence. In some lung tumors the activity of non-specific esterases was estimated biochemically (Table 2).

Positive immunofluorescence by itself is rather slender evidence; therefore we looked for further evidence of ACTH production. Of the 7 patients with positive ACTH fluorescence, 4 died and on 3 of these an autopsy was performed. All 3 patients exhibited hyperplasia of the adrenal cortex as in Cushing's disease. The clinician had suspected an ACTH-producing tumor in one patient, but rejected this possibility because the steroid excretion in the urine was in the high normal range. The other 3 patients are still alive.

Table 2. Activity of nonspecific esterases in lung tumors

Immunofluorescence method	Esterases
ACTH fluorescence	582 ± 166
no fluorescence	299 ± 61

On the basis of these four examples of enzyme histochemistry of human tumors:

— squamous-cell carcinoma of the lung
— adenocarcinoma of the endometrium
— carcinoma of the adrenal cortex
— ACTH-producing tumors,

we are able to discuss the relationship between enzyme activity and morphological and functional differentiation. As already stated, these are expressions of genetic information. In tumor cells we would expect enzyme activity to deviate from the morphological and functional differentiation. Only where the process of differentiation or function depends on the activity of an enzyme, should this deviation be impossible. The last situation is well demonstrated in enzyme histochemistry by carcinomas of the adrenal cortex, where hormone production is dependent on the activity of glucose-6-phosphate dehydrogenase and 3-beta-ol-steroid dehydrogenase.

In the three other examples given: keratinization of squamous-cell carcinomas of the lung, secretion in adenocarcinomas of the endometrium under progesterone treatment, and ACTH production in tumors, the dependence of these processes on the enzymes studied is not clear. As expected there is deviation between differentiation and enzyme activity in these tumors. The interesting point, however, in the first two of the above examples is that the enzyme activity gives a better indication of the degree of differentiation than the morphological aspects of the tumor cells. Thus, the activity of non-specific esterases correlates better with the prognosis of squamous-cell carcinoma of the lung than with the morphological differentiation of these tumors. In adenocarcinoma of the endometrium the changes in enzyme activity after treatment with progesterone derivatives are seen earlier and are more consistent than the morphological indications of secretion. In lung tumors which probably produce ACTH, the activity of esterases is correlated with this functional aspect.

Summary

In different human tumors the histochemically demonstrable activity of enzymes is correlated with morphological differentiation and hormone production. In squamous-cell carcinomas of the lung a distinct correlation between the activity of non-specific esterases and the biological behaviour as expressed in survival time after operation is proven. Adenocarcinomas of the endometrium show a decreased enzyme activity after prolonged treatment with progesterone derivatives. In adrenal cortex carcinomas seems to be a correlation between the functional differentiation and the activity of alkaline phosphatase. 7 of 50 lung tumors gave a positive immunofluorescence for ACTH. In 3 cases an autopsy could be performed, and all 3 exhibited hyperplasia of the adrenal cortex as in Cushing's syndrome.

References

FEYRTER, F.: Über die peripheren endokrinen (parakrinen) Drüsen des Menschen. Wien: Wilhelm Maudrich Verlag 1953.
PEARSE, A. G. E.: In: Calcitonin, proceedings of the symposium on thyrocalcitonin and the C cells. London: Heinemann 1967, p. 98.
PLANTEYDT, H. T., WILLIGHAGEN, R. G. J.: J. Path. Bact. **80**, 317 (1960).
PLANTEYDT, H. T., WILLIGHAGEN, R. G. J.: J. Path. Bact. **90**, 393 (1965).
THIERY, M., WILLIGHAGEN, R. G. J.: Amer. J. Obstet. Gynec. **95**, 1059 (1966).
THIERY, M., WILLIGHAGEN, R. G. J.: Amer. J. Obstet. Gynec. **99**, 173 (1967).
THIERY, M., WILLIGHAGEN, R. G. J.: Gynaecologia (Basel) **168**, 81 (1969).
WEG, R. A. VAN DE: Enzympatroon en functionele aktivität van de bijnierschors. Leiden: Thesis 1971.
WILLIGHAGEN, R. G. J.: In: Jaarboek van kankeronderzoek en kankerbestrijding **6**, 155 (1956).
WILLIGHAGEN, R. G. J., PLANTEYDT, H. T.: Nature (Lond.) **183**, 4653 (1959).
WILLIGHAGEN, R. G. J.: Nederl. T. Geneesk. **103**, 2522 (1959).
WILLIGHAGEN, R. G. J.: Jaarboek Kankerbestrijding **3**, 1803 (1960).
WILLIGHAGEN, R. G. J.: Ned. T. Geneesk. **105**, 1356 (1961).
WILLIGHAGEN, R. G. J.: Acta Histochem. suppl. **1961 II**, 177.
WILLIGHAGEN, R. G. J., VAN DER HEUL, R. O., VAN RIJSSEL, TH. G.: J. Path. Bact. **85**, 279 (1963).
WILLIGHAGEN, R. G. J.: Folia Histoch. Cytochem. **1**, 1 (1963).
WILLIGHAGEN, R. G. J., THIERY, M.: Amer. J. Obstet. Gynec. **100**, 393 (1968).
YOSHIMURA, Y., KAWANO, T., MORI, M.: Histochem. Meth. (München) **21**, 257 (1970).

Electron Microscopy of Oncocytomas and Carcinoid Tumors

H. SCHULZ

Numerous electron microscopical examinations of *oncocytes* and *oncocytomas* (HAMPERL, 1931, 1936), particularly of the salivary glands, have shown that oncocytes differ from other epithelial cells in their excessive proliferation of abnormal mitochondria (ROTH *et al.*, 1962; TANDLER and SHIPKEY, 1964; BALOGH and ROTH, 1965; MCGAVRAN, 1965; HÜBNER *et al.*, 1965; TANDLER, 1966; KLEINSASSER *et al.*, 1966; HÜBNER *et al.*, 1967). The cytoplasm is filled wither with numerous oval mitochondria, in which most of the cristae are stacked closely together in the center, or with longitudinal mitochondria having transverse tubular cristae (Fig. 1). Occa-

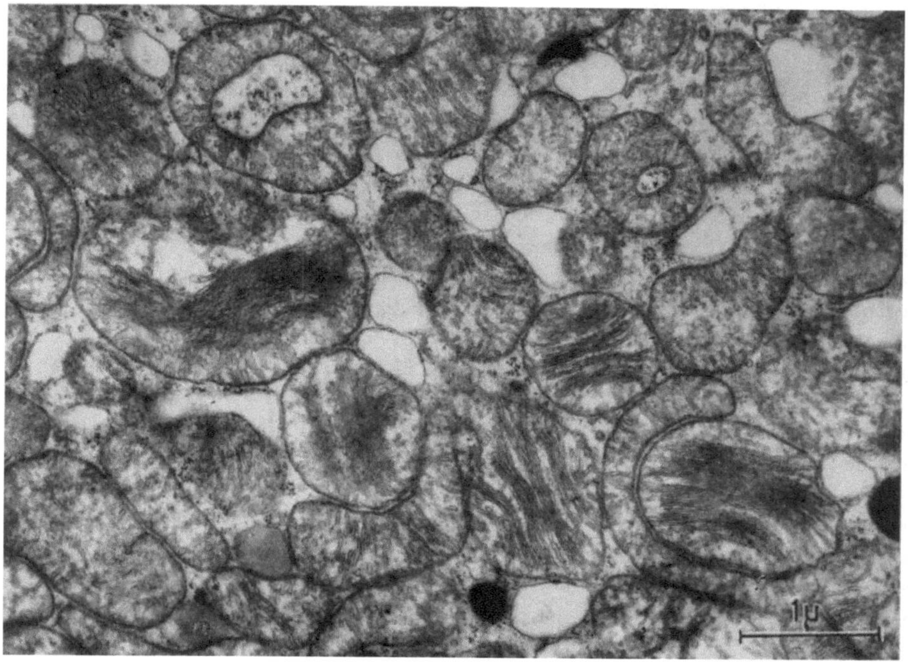

Fig. 1. Section of an oncocyte: cytoplasm densely populated by mitochondria which at time showed numerous closely packed cristae. Uranyl acetate. Electron microscope × 18,000. From P. BANNASCH, U. SCHACHT, R. WEIDNER u. E. STORCH, Verh. Dtsch. Ges. Path. **55**, 669 (1971)

sionally, the mitochondria of the oncocytomas contain aggregated glycogen. Mitochondria found in oncocytes are often larger than normal ones. Giant mitochondria are almost invariably spherical and sometimes have inner membranes arranged in arcade like layers, suggestive of Romanesque arches. Obviously, this special architectural structure of the inner membranes serves to make the giant mitochondria structurally more stable.

In the oxyphilic cells of the parathyroid and the Askanazy cells of the thyroid gland (TREMBLEY and PEARCE, 1960) histochemical examination, confirmed a distinctly increased activity of oxidative enzymes (FISCHER, 1961 and BALOGH and ROTH, 1965) also found a remarkable abundance of oxidative enzyme systems in oncocytic hyperplasia and oncocytomas of the thyroid gland, together with the histochemical absence of cytochrome oxidase and succinic dehydrogenase reactions. It appeared that the abundance of oxidases in the oncocytes was due to the increase of mitochondria as the carriers of these enzymes. In histochemical terms, oncocytes also give an enhanced phospholipid reaction and some increase in the activity of hydrolytic enzymes such as acid phosphatase and oc-naphthylacetate esterase (FISCHER and HÜBNER, 1969).

Experimentally it is possible to produce oncocyte tubuli and typical oncocytomas in the kidneys of rats treated with the carcinogen N-nitrosomorpholine (NMM). NMM-induced oncocytomas of rat kidney examined under the electron microscope again revealed the fine structure characteristic of oncocytes with hyperplasia of the chondriome (BANNASCH *et al.*, 1971). Intramitochondrial accumulation of glycogen, as found in some human oncocytomas (TANDLER *et al.*, 1970) was not seen in the NMM-induced oncocytomas. Since oncocytic adenomas and Hürthle-cell carcinomas of the human thyroid gland contain an abundance of oxidative enzyme systems in the Askanazy cells (TREMBLAY and PEARCE, 1960), they should not be regarded as degenerate but as efficiently functioning cells. Nevertheless, they are distinctly different in their function to normal thyroid cells. The enzyme systems required for the storage of iodine are missing in these cells and they are therefore unable to produce thyroid hormone (SOLLBERGER, 1957; WALTHARD, 1969), so that overstimulation or abnormal stimulation of the oncocytic epithelial cells of the thyroid gland may be assumed.

Recent results obtained by electron microscopy and histochemistry suggest that oncocytic transformation of the epithelial cells is certainly not a degenerative process. This transformation, in agreement with the original concept of HAMPERL (1931), should be regarded rather as a *re-differentiation* of epithelial cells, which develop an increased but unbalanced metabolic activity. However, FISCHER and HÜBNER (1969) have shown that oncocytic cells do not invariably have greater functional efficiency.

In order to find out why the mitochondria increase in number, SCHIEFER *et al.* (1968), and HÜBNER and SCHIEFER (1968), isolated oncocytic giant mitochondria from adenolymphomas. They found a reduced P/O quotient and a very loose connection between respiration and oxidative phosphorylation in the isolated oncocyte mitochondria. However, the cytochrome spectra and lipoid analyses did not deviate substantially from those of the mitochondria of other organs and other species. Although the mitochondria of the oncocytes do not have any electron-dense matrix inclusions containing Ca^{++}, they nevertheless take up large amounts of calcium when placed in a medium containing Ca^{++}, in the same way as normal mitochondria.

Unlike normal mitochondria, however, oncocyte mitochondria produce only very small quantities of high-energy phosphate (ATP). The conditions prevailing are much the same as those in brown adipose tissue, which also contains a large number of mitochondria and serves for chemical thermo-regulation. The functional defect of the oncocyte mitochondria thus takes the form of a mitochondriopathy (HÜBNER, 1971). Apparently, the oncocytes attempt to compensate for this functional defect by providing a greater number of mitochondria and substantially increasing the surface area of the mitochondria membranes. This leads to hypertrophy and hyperplasia of the chondriome. Oncocytic transformation must therefore be regarded as the consequence of an acquired disturbance of the mitochondrial enzyme organization. As oncocytes are able to divide, their pathological metabolic activity is passed on to the daughter cells.

Carcinoids are relatively rare epithelial tumors which favour the intestinal tract, particularly in the region of the small intestine and appendix. Carcinoids may also metastasize in the regional lymph nodes and in other organs of the abdominal cavity and can cause the so-called flush syndrome.

Carcinoids develop from the enterochromaffine cells (GOSSET and MASSON, 1914; FEYRTER, 1934) which produce a vasoactive substance: 5-hydroxytryptamine (5-HT). According to RATZENHOFER and LEMBECK (1954) 5-HT is associated with the granula of the carcinoid cells. BULLÓN-RAMÎREZ *et al.* (1960) and WETZSTEIN *et al.* (1962) described the ultrastructure and the electron microscopical histochemistry of the enterochromaffine cells and their specific granula found in the duodenum of the guinea pig. WOOD (1965) found a positive reaction of the granula in enterochromaffine cells of the rat duodenum, after incubation in 2.5% potassium dichromate solution. He concluded that potassium-dichromate was suitable for the determination of unsubstituted catecholamines. FORSSMANN *et al.* (1969) recognized five types of enterochromaffine cells, and assumed that each type had a separate endocrine function: Cell type I was responsible for the production of 5-HT, type II cells were comparable to the A-cells and type III to the D-cells of the pancreas islets. Cell type IV was claimed to be responsible for the production of catecholamines, and type V for gastrin. RUBIN *et al.* (1971), however, carried out a combination of autoradiographical and electron microscopical studies and found that almost all the various types of endocrine cells in the gastric mucosal membrane of the mouse, and the granula of its mastocytes were able to bind labelled 5-hydroxytryptophan (5-HTP). The radioactive labelling was limited to the specific granula of the cytoplasm. LANGER (1960, 1961) stated that the bronchial carcinoid differed from that of the small intestine by the fact that osmiophilic granula were not present in the former.

The bronchial carcinoid is a solid adenoma, the cells of which are characterized by their high degree of differentiation. BOUTEILLE *et al.* (1964) unlike LANGER (1961) found in six bronchial carcinoids specific granula with a diameter of 150 microns. It was possible to demonstrate the specific presence of unsubstituted catecholamines and indolamines in the granula cytochemically by means of the glutaraldehyde-dichromate reaction. After fixation with glutaraldehyde VERLEY (1965) also found numerous specific secretory granules in carcinoid tumors of the bronchus, these granules being similar to those present in normal argentaffin cells and carcinoid tumors of the digestive tract.

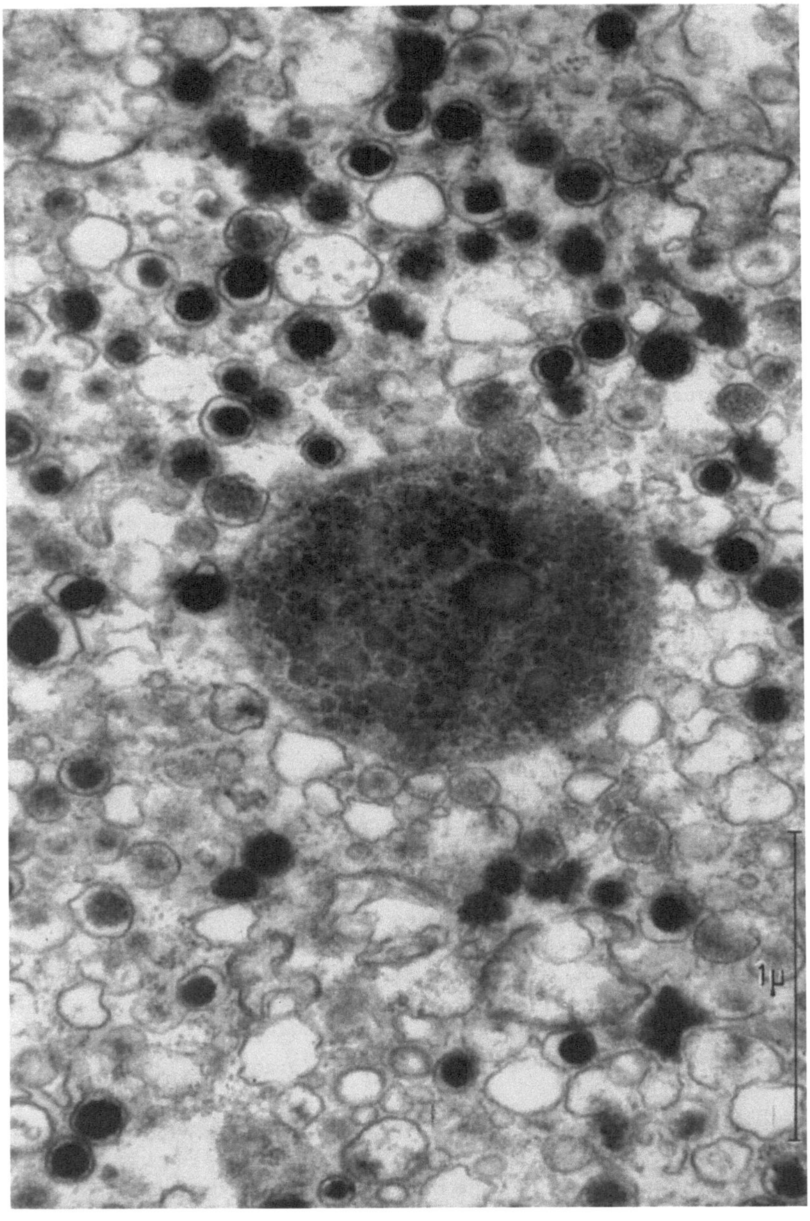

Fig. 2. Carcinoid of the small intestine from a 62-year old male. Section of the cytoplasm of a cell of the primary tumor. Specific serotonin granule; in the center of the figure is a granular cytosome (lyosome). Arch. no. 3415 D/63 Electron microscope × 11,300. Final magnification × 42,100. From. A. SCHUMACHER and H. SCHULZ, Klin. Wschr. **41**, 1191 (1963)

SCHUMACHER and SCHULZ (1963) examined a primary carcinoid of the small intestine and metastases in the lymph node. They applied histochemical methods at the electron microscopical level to investigate the endocrine efficiency ratings associated with certain cell structures. In addition, they tested tumor cell fractions of lymph node metastases for their serotonin content and carried out comparative electron microscopical studies of the tumor cell fractions. The cytoplasm of the tumor cells contained numerous, round to oval, specific granula, which were surrounded by a light halo and enclosed by a membrane (Fig. 2). The degree of osmiophily and the electron density of the specific granula varied. The average diameter of the long and short axes were $d_{max} = 181$ microns and $d_{min} = 141$ microns. The diameter of the round homogenous, osmiophilic contents of the granula averaged 106 microns. The abundance of specific granula at the edges of the tumor cell complexes was identical to the distribution of the diffuse, granular and strong fluorescence, and the argentaffinity of the histochemical reactions. Granular lysosomes were also found in the tumor cells. They tended to occur primarily near the nucleus and were also fluorescent and argentaffin. The cell nuclei of intestinal carcinoid tumors were usually round, and when observed under the electron microscope showed an equal distribution of the chromoplasm and a distinctly visible nucleolus. Frequently the perinuclear space was much larger than normal and there were numerous nuclear pores. The ergastoplasm was wide-meshed and the numerous mitochondria, which were usually small in size, had normal inner structures. In the smallest particle fractions, the tumor cell fractions were characterized by a substantially higher content of serotonin than usual. The total serotonin content of the tumor was 473 μg wet weight in the metastasis. At the electron microscopical level the specific granula of carcinoid tumors were very similar to the specific cell elements of a number of endocrine organs, such as the pheochrome granula of the suprarenal medulla, the granula of A-cells and B-cells in islets of the pancreas, the neuro-secretory elementary granula, the specific granulations of the cells of the anterior lobe of the hypophysis, and the granula of the calcitonin-producing C-cells of the thyroid gland.

Summary

Oncocytes and *oncocytomas* are caused by a functional and structural anomaly of the mitochondria which, according to electron microscopical findings, induces an excessive increase in the number of mitochondria and greatly enlarges the surface of the mitochondrial membranes. In biochemical terms this mitochondiopathy results, to a large extent, in the decoupling of respiration and oxidative phosphorylation. The oncocytic cell transformation which occurs with increasing age in numerous glandular organs, and which can be provoked experimentally in animals by N-nitrosomorpholine, is based on a generally valid pathogenetic principle and is brought about by the unbalanced metabolism of secreting epithelial cells.

Carcinoid tumors originate from enterochromaffine cells and are usually endocrinologically active. Radioactive labelling experiments have established that 5-hydroxytryptamine (5-HT) is localized in specific granula, 140—180 microns in diameter, in the cytoplasm of the carcinoid cells. Under the electron microscope the specific granula of carcinoid cells look very similar to the specific cytoplasmic granula of a number of other endocrine organs.

References

BALOGH, K., ROTH, S. I.: Lab. Invest. **14**, 310 (1965).
BANNASCH, P., SCHACHT, U., WEIDNER, R., STORCH, E.: Verh. dtsch. Ges. Path. **55**, 665 (1971).
BOUTEILLE, M., ABELANET, R., DELARUE, J.: Ann. Anat. path. **9**, 398 (1964).
BULLÓN-RAMÍREZ, A., LANGER, E., SCHULZ, H.: Rev. clín. esp. **5**, 321 (1960).
FEYRTER, F.: Ergebn. allg. Path. path. Anat. **29**, 305 (1934).
FISCHER, R.: Virchows Arch. Abt. A Path. Anat. **334**, 445 (1961).
FISCHER, R., HÜBNER, G.: Histochemie und Feinstruktur der Onkozyten. Manuskript: Wissenschaftliche Sitzung am 13. 12. 1969 in Bonn anläßlich des 70. Geburtstages von Prof. Dr. Dr. h. c. H. Hamperl.
FORSSMANN, W. G, ORCI, L., PICTET, R., RENOLD, A. E., ROUILLER, C.: J. Cell. Biol. **40**, 692 (1969).
GOSSET, A., MASSON, P.: Presse méd. **22**, 237 (1914).
HAMPERL, H.: Virchows Arch. Abt. A Path. Anat. **282**, 724 (1931).
HAMPERL, H.: Virchows Arch. Abt. A Path. Anat. **298**, 327 (1936).
HAMPERL, H.: Virchows Arch. Abt. A Path. Anat. **300**, 46 (1937).
HAMPERL, H.: Virchows Arch. Abt. A Path. Anat. **335**, 452 (1962 a).
HAMPERL, H.: Z. Krebsforsch. **64**, 427 (1962 b).
HÜBNER, G.: Hals-, Nas.- u. Ohrenarzt, **19**, 137 (1971).
HÜBNER, G., KLEIN, H. J., SCHÜMMELFEDER N.: Klin. Wschr. **43**, 798 (1965).
HÜBNER, G., PAULUSSEN, F., KLEINSASSER, O.: Virchows Arch. Abt. A Path. Anat. **343**, 34 (1967).
HÜBNER, G., SCHIEFER, H.: Excerpta Medica, Interat. Congr. Ser. No. 166, XIIth International Congress of Cell Biology, Brussels, Abstract **88**, August 25 (1968).
KLEINSASSER, O., KLEIN, H. J., STEINBACH, E., HÜBNER, G.: Arch. klin. exp. Ohr.-Nas. u. Kehlk.-Heilk. **186**, 317 (1966).
LANGER, E.: Verh. dtsch. Ges. Path. **44**, 267 (1960).
LANGER, E.: In: Symposium über Krebsprobleme. Berlin-Göttingen-Heidelberg: Springer 1961.
MC GAVRAN, M. H.: Virchows Arch. Abt. A Path. Anat. **338**, 195 (1965).
RATZENHOFER, M., LEMBECK, F.: Z. Zellforsch. **60**, 169 (1954).
ROTH, I. S., OLEN, E., HANSEN, S. L.: Lab. Invest. **11**, 933 (1962).
RUBIN, W., GERSHON, M. D., ROSS, L. L.: J. Cell. Biol. **50**, 399 (1971).
SCHIEFER, H.-G., HÜBNER, G., KLEINSASSER, O.: Virchows Arch. Abt. B Zellpath. **1**, 230 (1968).
SCHUMACHER, A., SCHULZ, H.: Klin. Wschr. **41**, 1188 (1963).
SOLLBERGER, W.: Schweiz. Z. Path. **20**, 286 (1957).
TANDLER, B.: Arch. Otolaryng. **84**, 90 (1966).
TANDLER, B., HUTTER, R. V. P., ERLANDSON, R. A.: Lab. Invest. **23**, 567 (1970).
TANDLER, B., SHIPKEY, F. H.: J. Ultrastruct. Res. **11**, 292 (1964).
TREMBLAY, G., PEARCE, A. G. E.: J. Path. Bact. **80**, 353 (1960).
VERLEY, J. M.: Z. Krebsforsch. **66**, 503 (1965).
WALTHARD, B.: In: Spezielle path. Anat. **4**, 321 (1969).
WETZSTEIN, R., DOERFLER, W., SCHWINK, A.: Protoplasma (Wien) **55**, 303 (1962).
WOOD, J. G.: Tex. Rep. Biol. Med. **23**, 828 (1965).

The Histology of Rare Human Tumors and their Relationships to General Tumor Pathology

R. LAUMONIER and G. CHOMETTE

Certain human tumors may be considered rare in the light of certain facts:

— the low percentage rate of certain cancers leads to a rare statistical level amongst tumors in general. This rarity is absolute for certain very rare cancers in all countries, and for all workers (such as the esthésioneurocytoma). It is relative for certain geographical distributions (hepatomas) and for age (example: adult nephroblastoma).

— the morphological rarity is represented by the fact that some relatively rare tumors sometimes show unusual histological aspects. These may be undifferentiated forms of usually differentiated cancers (anaplastic forms of ostéogenic sarcomas), or unusual differentiations (rare épidermoid carcinomas of the stomach). This group is the main supply of Nadal Masson's "ignotomas" which are the concern and sometimes the confusion of pathologists (MASSON 1968).

— the rarity of their evolution is shown by the disconcerting behaviour of certain tumors with regard to their natural history. Either cancers which do not generally give rise to secondaries, develop visceral metastasis (such as the basal cell carcinoma of the skin). Or, an abnormally long evolution is found in patients with a very malignant tumor (melanomas, generalized carcinomas). Or, even spontaneous recovery is found (choriocarcinoma of the placenta, rare observations of glandular carcinomas).

There are variable relationships between these different concepts of rarity and the general pathology of tumors, which should be examined in comparison with three pathological principals:

- the carcinogenic stimulus,
- the proliferation of tumor clones,
- the reactions of the host organism.

— The cancerogenic stimuli intervene as a factor of statistical rarity: so that rare, abnormal genotypes correspond to rare varieties of tumors.

— The elective proliferation of certain clones influences the morphological and evolutive rarities.

— The reactions of the host organism condition rare or unusual developments, as well as unfrequent morphological aspects.

These relationships are thus shown:

Stimulus	——→	Statistical rarity
Clone	——→	Morphological rarity
Reaction of the host organism	——→	Developmental rarity (Rarity of evolution)

a) Rare and precise carcinogenic stimuli represent the statistical rarity of certain tumors. The hereditary trait is well shown in the retinoblastoma, congenital multiple polyposis of the colon, the syndrome of Peutz Jeghers, and also for certain phacomatosis. There is either a genotype abnormality without an abnormal caryotype, or a caryotype abnormality (the incidence of acute leucemias in mongols).

— Pleural mesotheliomas are rare tumors: their relation to asbestosis forms an even smaller group. Also aminotumors are rare in the bladder carcinoma group.

— Very rare but well-known are the sarcomas which develop in the irradiated cancer tissue.

— Bilharzia bladder papillomas, and the association of parasites and cancer in general (cancer of the cervix and bilharzia) are rare in non-endemic countries. The role of viruses in human pathology is one of the perspective principals of cancer research. The african hematosarcoma may be an approach to this problem.

b) The morphological rarity, and to a certain extent the developmental rarity, of different tumors are the consequence of the proliferation of an unusual cell clone.

One may take different types of clones as examples. Some proliferate from *embryological structures*. Blastomas tumors are, amongst tumors in general, rare (whether they be neuroblastomas, renal blastomas or genital blastomas). The balance between the undifferentiation of the cellular mass and the tendency more or less clear cut to differentiation explain some even more rare aspects (renal blastomas to cartilaginous, muscular part, PAYAN 1971). In dysembryonas which are not uncommon tumors, one may be surprised to find structures corresponding to the first 15 days of embryogenesis, in the form of embryological fragments, blastocytes with two vesicules (PEYRON 1941 a et b).

Other rare clones come from *adult tissues*. First it must be noted that certain cells never arise from tumor clones (Paneth cells) and that certain cancers only develop very rarely from certain tissues (carcinoma of the small intestine). It may therefore be supposed that certain cell families, which are highly differentiated, are unadapted to neoplastic proliferation, and that certain rare tumors develop from the proliferation of contingent cells which are normally present in the tissue matrix but little disposed to hyperplasia (parafollicular cells and medullary carcinomas of the thyroïd).

Other rare tumor clones arising from adult tissues proliferate to take up embryological properties: this is so in α-foetoprotein producing hepatomas. This property is also seen in certain embryological tumors and very rarely in carcinomas of general morphology with secondaries in the liver. The origin of these foetoproteins from liver tumors has been discussed. (It may be the "foetal" regression of proliferating tumor hepatocytes, or hyperplasia of residual embryological cells, or properties of the regenerating liver?) It is interesting to note that the study of Feulgen positive material shows the monoclonal "infantile" character of certain adult hepatomas

(LAUMONIER 1963) which may be an argument in favour of the origin of these clones from embryonic cell fragments.

The rarity of other adult clones is connected with changes in their productive properties in comparison with their tissue matrix. Sometimes the ordinary secretion of this type of cell is missing (non-secreting carcinoid tumors of the rectum). Sometimes properties of secretion appear in cell clones which are not normally secreting (hypoglycemia producing by mesenchymomas). Certain rare tumors owe the uncertainty of their origin to these changes in their histological properties: myoid tumors of the stomach are an example.

The understanding of these clonal deviation may be facilitated by several notions of tissue organogenesis.

First, there are the "cell systems" of Feyrter and the tissue planes (trophopigmentary planes of BORREL), which explain certain rare tumor associations: multivisceral adenomas, phacomatosis, neurocutaneous melanosis (DAILLY 1965) (Fig. 1).

Secondly, the notion of anatomical regions corresponds to the unequal evolution of tumors of the same structure (melanoblastomas). Here is placed the unusual affinity of certain tumors for certain tissues (lymph node secondaries tumors of alveolar rhabdomyosarcomas of Riopelle).

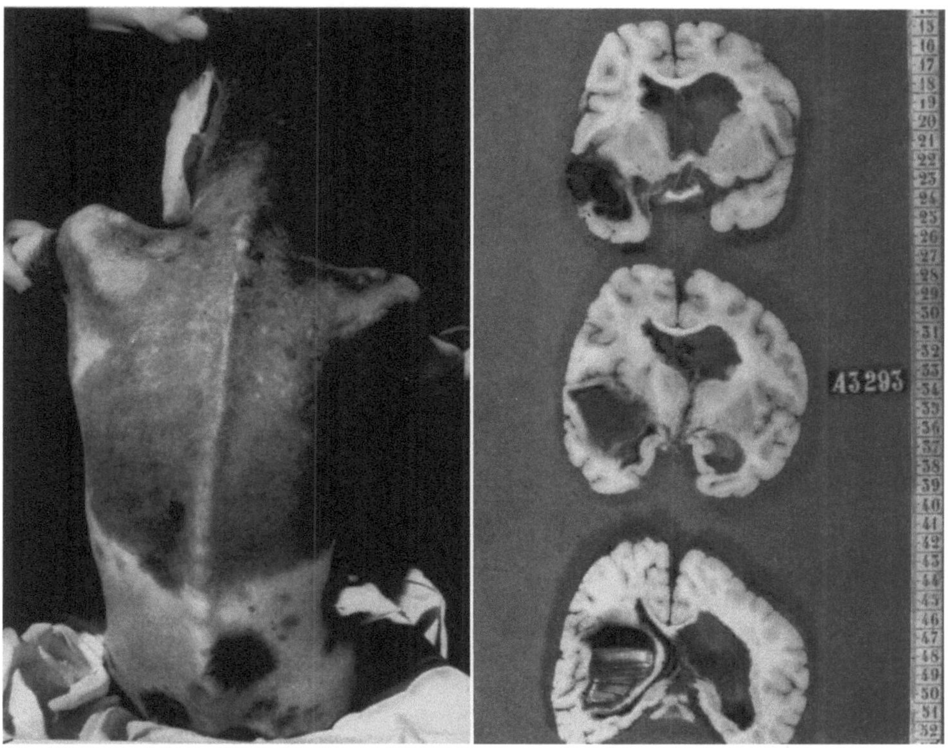

Fig. 1 a and b. Neurocutaneal melanosis, a benign giant naevus "in cape", b meningo-encephalic malignant melanoma

Third, there is the notion of tissue organisers. The old embryological theory is still up to date. Certain work, such as that of Saxen, shows the effect of reciprocal induction of metanephrotic mesenchyme and of the ureteral Wolffen bud. This effect is changed by adding filters. It may be seen that there is a disorder in the blastomas developed in the mature organism and not in the embryon. Amongst the tissue organiser, it may be seen that when a part of an embryon is grafted, the fragments which live and develop are irrigated by the host. "The complexity of the embryon is therefore a function of its initial vascularisation" (Masson). This notion of organisers and of vascular systems helps to explain the morphological and developmental rarity of some "adult" cell clones: the smallest tumors already possess this vascular system (in some experimental cancerogenic processes the vascular changes go before the clone proliferation: the melanoma of the Hamster). The system may be delicate, leading to certain unexpected developments (Fig. 2) (Delarue 1965). This is so in small carcinomas which develop in polyps of the colon; when the polyp falls off its pedicle by necrosis, there is not necessarly a renewal of the cancerogenic process.

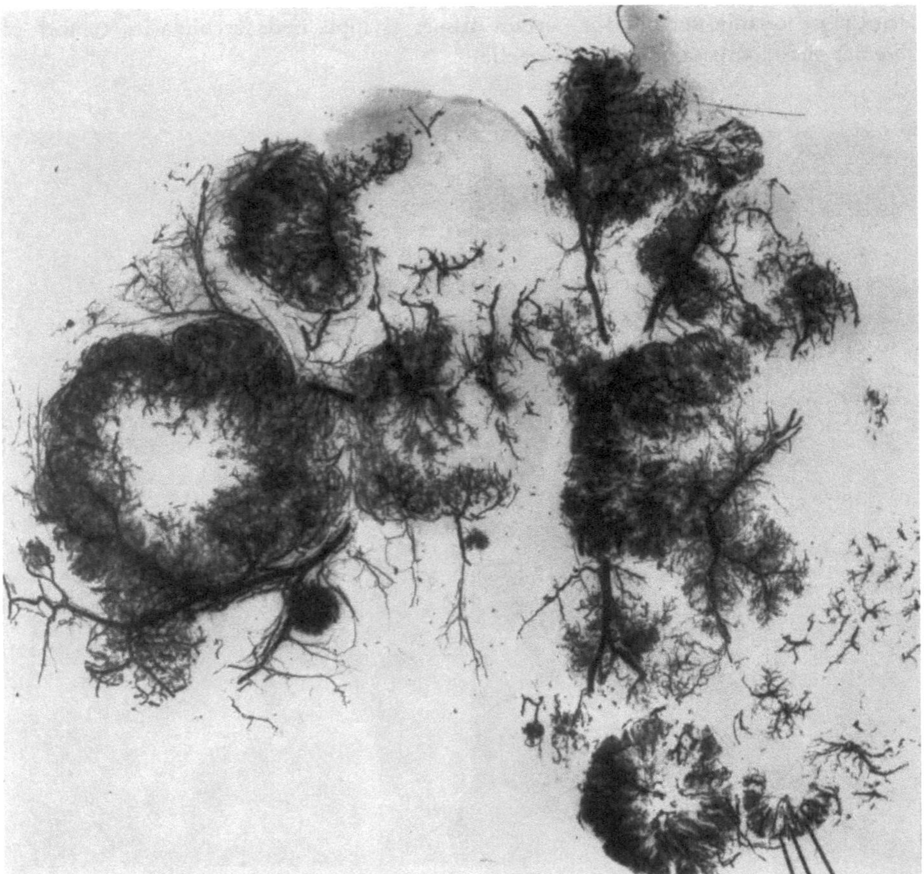

Fig. 2. Hepatic metastases: vascular tufts at the periphery of each metastasis

These notions of vascularisation organisers fit into a larger setting of relationships between host and tumor.

c) The modalities of the reactions of the host make up another approach to the concept of tumor rarity. Two groups of facts should be distinguished:

Firstly, the secretions and the properties of the neoplastic clones can induce certain morphological changes in the host, such as in stromal amyloidosis in medullary carcinomas of the thyroïd; and as in calcospherites of papillary carcinomas. It is also true for the hyperelastogenesis of mesenteric arterioles which correspond to carcinoïd tumors (ANTHONY, 1970). Fibroblastic modifications of certain tumors belong also to this group. This may be either the simultaneous proliferation of epithelial and mesenchymatous clones in very rare carcinosarcomas of the thyroid which are in actual fact more often blastoma tumors of a particular kind (müllerblastoma of the body of the uterus).

Or, this may be a special modification on the fibroblasts in contact with the epithelial tumor: the fibroepithelioma of Pinkus develops as a basal cell carcinoma. Or it may finally be that the action of the mesenchyme confers upon the tumor its rarity at the same time as its very unusual development (SPÄRCK 1969): this is so for phylloid tumors of the breast of which we are presenting an unusual observation in two sisters.

In a second group of facts, the histological changes show the defence reaction of the host against the clone proliferation. This may be seen in lymphoïd stroma carcinomas (medullary carcinoma of the breast which has a better evolution than other breast cancers). It may also to seen in the tuberculoïd histiocyte hyperplasia of satellite lymph nodes without secondaries — (in some gastric, biliary and cervical

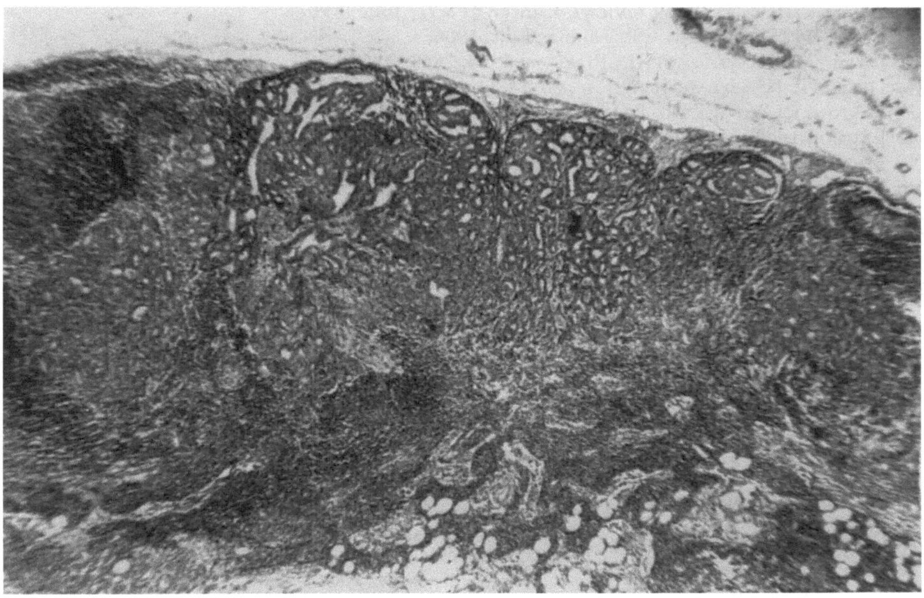

Fig. 3. Lymph node: metastasis of pancreatic carcinoma (Icterus — choledocho-enterostomy; the patient is always living after fifteen years)

uterine carcinomas). All this is the scope of tumor immunology. Since the discovery of FOLEY in 1952, we know with certainty that experimental cancer cells carry neoantigens KLEIN in 1966 identified a neoantigen of human tumor in the african hematosarcoma.

The choriocarcinoma is an example of a rare tumor from every point of view (*statistical:* $^{1}/_{40\,000}$ pregnancies, in France *morphological* because the usual criteria of invasion, destruction and atypical reaction are not valid for it (ELSTON 1969), *developmental* because recovery may be obtained by anti-mitotic drug therapy associated with surgery in half the cases, and involution or recovery may take place spontaneously). This is an example of a grafted tumor which brings about immunological processes (MATHÉ 1967, AMIEL 1967). It is the best example of spontaneous regression of cancers.

This question has already been raised (see the papers of BOYD in 1966 and ASHWORTH in 1967). Even with the incompromising notes of Ashworth, it is possible to bring together all the uncontestable facts and we have brought some examples to show this (Fig. 3).

The identification of antigens, at first the sphere of immunochemists, may become the realm of immunohistiochemists. Thus the improvements in histology will bring about a better understanding of tumor rarities and so of tumors in general, and will help "to find the answer to the enigmas which one set repeatedly by the fertile invention of illness" (MASSON).

References

1. AMIEL, J. L.: In: Cell bound immunity, 143, p. 197, Liège 1967.
2. ANTHONY, P. P., DRURY, R. A.: J. clin. Path. **23**, 110 (1970).
3. ASHWORTH, C. T.: Book reviews, Cancer Res. **27**, 1007 (1967).
4. BOYD, W.: Springfield: CT. Thomas Edit. 1966.
5. DAILLY, R., FORTHOMME, J.: Presse méd. **73**, 2867 (1965).
6. DELARUE, J., ABELANET, A., CHOMETTE, G.: Presse méd. **73**, 1517 (1965).
7. ELSTON, C. W.: J. Path. Bact. **97**, 261 (1969).
8. LAUMONIER, R., LAQUERRIERE, R., MARCHE, C.: Rev. franç. Etud. clin. biol. **8**, 884 (1963).
9. MASSON, P.: Paris: Maloine Edit. 1968.
10. MATHE, G.: Bull. Cancer **58**, 33 (1967).
11. PAYAN, A.: Arch. Anat. path. **19**, 153, (1971).
12. PEYRON, A.: C. R. Soc. Biol. (Paris) **135**, 281 (1941).
13. PEYRON, A.: C. R. Soc. Biol. (Paris) **135**, 347 (1941).
14. SPÄRCK, J. V.: Acta path. microbiol. scand. **77**, 24 (1969)

Chromosome Changes in Human Malignant Tumors: An Evaluation

A. A. Sandberg

It appears extremely unlikely that visual microscopy, including the application of new techniques such as that of fluorescent staining [7] and the determination of the "banding" patterns of human chromosomes [4, 40], will yield in the near future any characteristic or specific cytogenetic finding similar to that of the Ph^1-chromosome in chronic myelocytic leukemia (CML) [38]. The description of the latter by Nowell and Hungerford [38] remains a singular milestone in the field of medical oncology and cytogenetics. Hence, this paper will deal with an assessment and evaluation of published chromosomal findings in human leukemia and cancer as these bear upon:

1. Specificity of karyotypic alterations in human neoplasia,
2. The role of chromosomal changes (including "markers") in the causation of human cancer and leukemia, and
3. Possible future application of cytogenetic data in the diagnosis and treatment of these diseases.

Before these three areas are discussed, it may be appropriate to present a view regarding some of the features of the human genome and how these may be related to the evolution of cytogenetic changes in human neoplasia.

The human genome is a fragile thing, tending to undergo an array of structural changes in its chromosomes, i. e., breakages, gap formation, rearrangements, fragmentations, translocations, etc., when exposed *in vitro* to almost any biologic, chemical or physical agent. Even though there may be a difference, both quantitative and qualitative, in the susceptibility to such changes with the tissue origin of the cells, and this may apply both to *in vitro* and *in vivo* conditions, almost all cells will manifest cytogenetic alterations when exposed to exogenous agents (Fig. 1). In fact, under tissue culture conditions human cells may undergo profound karyotypic alterations without any apparent exogenous agent being implicated [46, 58], though it is possible that the biologic ecology of the culture may have changed [12] and, thus, resulted in the chromosomal aberrations. Even though it has not been documented as profusely *in vivo* as under *in vitro* conditions, there is every likelihood that the human genome is just as susceptible to damage by external and internal substances *in vivo* as *in vitro*. In all probability the stochastic karyotypic changes observed *in vitro*, when cells are exposed to noxious agents, may also occur *in vitro*, though they are observed more readily in the former state due to our failure and inability to examine cells *in vivo* containing these fleeting and unstable chromosomal aberrations.

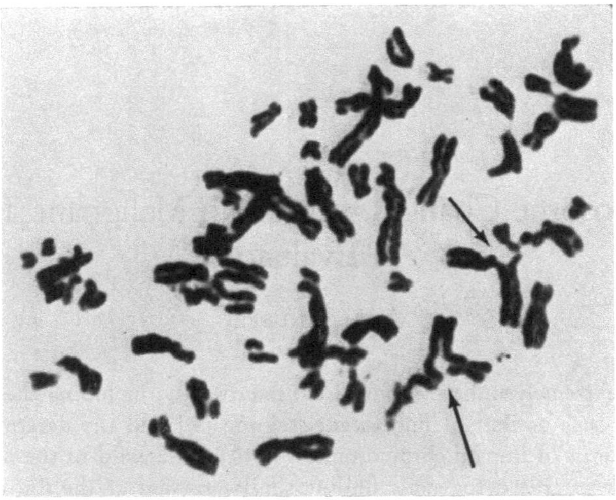

Fig. 1. Metaphase of a marrow cell from a patient with acute leukemia who had developed measles and showed chromosomal aberrations in his blood and marrow cell for over one year. Arrows point to extremely aberrant units

Under *in vitro* conditions and, particularly, *in vivo* almost all of the cells with profound and multiple chromosomal changes are ultimately eliminated. However, it is possible that through a process of selection, some of the cells containing cytogenetic abnormalities, be they morphological or numerical, may survive and actually gain growth potential exceeding that of the normal diploid cells [20]. It is this type of process which may ultimately lead to the overgrowth of the normal diploid cells *in vitro* by aneuploid cells or to the genesis of aneuploid cancer cells which may invade and infiltrate normal tissues.

What is the evidence that cellular events, such as those just described, do occur *in vivo* and lead to the development of cancer or leukemia in human subjects? Obviously, changes in the genome cannot be monitored as closely or frequently (and often not all) *in vivo* as *in vitro* and, hence, resort has to be made to an analysis and interpretation of data obtained on premalignant, early malignant, and non-invasive lesions in humans, as they relate to the role of cytogenetic changes in the genesis of neoplasia. The best sources of such materials are lesions of the uterine cervix [1, 3, 8, 25, 56] and benign tumors of the brain and intestine (particularly polyps) [29—31]. In truly benign lesions of these areas, the cytogenetic picture is invariably diploid [29, 31, 33, 63]. The karyotypic changes which have been observed under "mildly" abnormal conditions, such as cervical dysplasia or changes in the histology of colonic polyps, have consisted of a wide array of chromosomal aberrations, very much resembling those induced by noxious agents in cultured lymphocytes *in vitro*. These remarkable cytogenetic changes have shown no specific picture or characteristic chromosomal change for any lesion. In time, of course, some of the involved cells containing more stable chromosomal changes, be they numerical and/or morphological, may become apparent in these lesions, though this tends to occur with further entrenchment and progression of the neoplastic process. As the latter gains the upper hand in the tissue of origin, the tumor usually settles on a characteristic karyotype which, however, differs from one tumor to another, even in the same tissue of origin. The karyotype thus selected appears to endow the tumor with unusual growth and metastasizing potential. In essence, what was just described is the "clonal" evolution of human neoplasia [6, 10, 11, 60], a hypothesis which does not differ basically from the "stem cell" concept advanced by MAKINO [32] and some of his predecessors regarding chromosomes and neoplasia [50].

1. Specificity of Karyotypic Alterations in Human Neoplasia

The only consistent, characteristic and relatively specific cytogenetic finding in human neoplasia remains the Ph^1-chromosome in chronic myelocytic leukemia [10, 18, 19, 49, 53]. The application of fancy (and sometimes not so fancy) statistical and computer analysis to karyotypic data in human cancer and leukemia [1, 8, 13, 27, 35, 37, 55, 57], in order to implicate this or that groups of chromosomes as related to the genesis of these diseases, has not withstood the test of common cytogenetic sense and careful analysis [43, 47]. That in some tissues or under certain conditions one group of chromosomes may be more frequently involved than another may only be related to the already alluded to differences in susceptibility of the chromosomes among cells of different tissue origin. The lack of cytogenetic consistency from case to case, and often in the cells of the same tumor, mitigates against the changes in one or another group of chromosomes as being causally involved in any particular tumor. Nevertheless, some generalizations regarding chromosomes in human cancer and leukemia can be made:

A. Human acute leukemia is accompanied by a normal chromosome number and distribution in at least 50% of the cases [43, 45, 48, 49, 50].

a) Acute lymphoblastic leukemia (preponderantly the acute leukemia of children) is almost invariably associated with pseudo- or hyperdiploidy and, sometimes, very high ploidy (Fig. 2), when chromosomal changes are present in this disease.

b) Acute myeloblastic leukemia may be associated with hypo-, pseudo- or hyperdiploidy, the abnormal chromosome number, however, almost never exceeding 55.

c) Fuzziness and ill-definition of the chromosomes, even in diploid metaphases, is a frequent observation in leukemic cells af acute leukemia [24, 43, 45, 48] and deserves further attention of investigators, since the mechanism responsible for this is unknown.

d) "Marker" chromosomes do not occur frequently in the cells of acute leukemia; however, see the discussion about "marker" chromosomes below, in order to fully understand this fact of cytogenetic changes in leukemia.

B. The preponderant number (100%?) of human cancers has been found to be accompanied by chromosomal changes and these range from severe hypodiploidy to remarkable hyperploidy (Fig. 3) [1, 9, 29, 49, 50, 56, 62].

a) No characteristic or specific karyotypic picture has emerged for any tumor and no 2 tumors with identical karyotypes have been described, to-date.

b) Diploid cancers have been described, though they are very rare [9]. Nevertheless, the occurrence of such tumors indicates that diploidy and neoplasia are compatible.

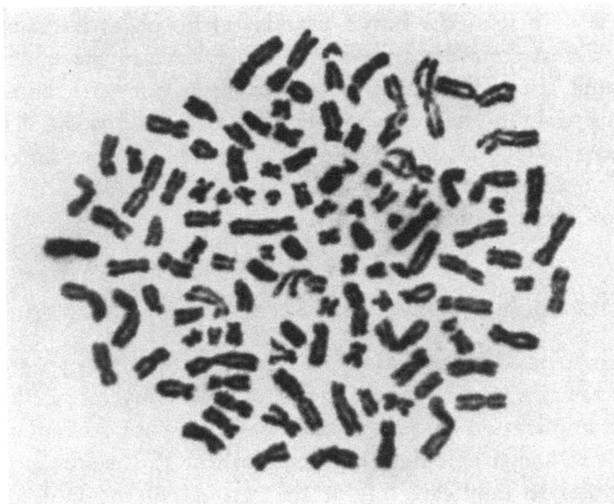

Fig. 2. A metaphase of modal marrow cells from a patient with acute lymphoblastic leukemia containing an extremely large number of chromosomes (more than 90). The various chromosomes could be assigned to various karyotypic groups of the human karyotype. Many of the chromosomes, particularly the metacentric and submetacentric ones, could readily be abnormal "marker" chromosomes and escape detection, due to their resemblance to normal chromosomes

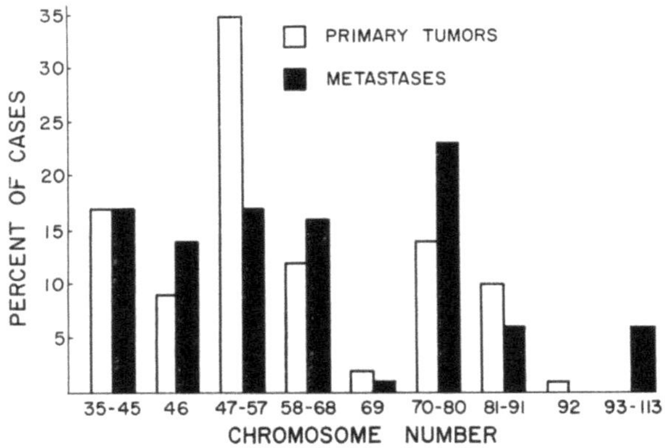

Fig. 3. Distribution of the percentage of cancers observed in our laboratory (primary, 151 cases and metastatic, 222 cases), with different chromosome modal numbers. The euploid cells (diploid = 46; triploid = 69; tetraploid = 92) contained abnormal distributions of chromosomes and were, in fact, pseudoeuploid

c) "Marker" chromosomes are very frequent in human cancers and their metastases, egregiously abnormal chromosomes being found in at least 50% of the cancers.

C. The Ph[1]-chromosome is consistently and caracteristically found in the cells of chronic myelocytic leukemia (CML) [18].

a) When chronic myelocytic leukemia undergoes blastic transformation, the Ph^1-chromosome usually persists in the cells and may, in fact, double or triple in some cases.

b) Other chromosomal changes, usually consisting of hyperdiploidy, may herald or accompany the development of the blastic phase of chronic myelocytic leukemia. When this phase responds to therapy, which is rather rare, the karyotypic aberrations in the hyperdiploid cells may disappear, though the Ph^1-chromosome usually persists.

c) To-date, no Ph^1-negative cases of CML have been shown to become Ph^1-positive and this probably also applies to the reversed condition, i. e., no Ph^1-positive case has been shown, with any definitiveness, to become Ph^1-negative.

d) The Ph^1-chromosome may occur in conditions other than chronic myelocytic leukemia [19], though these conditions are usually closely allied to CML (e. g., acute myeloblastic leukemia, polycythemia vera, erythremic myelosis, etc.). However, the Ph^1-chromosome has been described in two probable cases of acute lymphoblastic leukemia [41, 52].

2. The Role of Chromosomal Changes (Including "Markers") in the Causation of Human Cancer and Leukemia

The role of chromosomal changes in the initial and direct causation of human cancer and leukemia has been exhaustively reviewed and argued about and remains a problem that is far from being settled [17, 20, 28, 32, 43]. We are of the rather strong view that the chromosomal changes in human neoplasia are epiphenomena secondary to the neoplastic process and are not directly involved in the initial causation of the neoplastic state. The only exception may be the Ph^1-chromosome in chronic myelocytic leukemia, though even here there are certain facts that do not entirely support the view of the abnormal chromosome playing a pristine role in the development of the leukemia [49].

Besides the fact that only about 50% of human acute leukemias are accompanied by aneuploidy in the leukemic cells and that cases which are aneuploid tend to show different karyotypes from case to case without any consistent abnormalities, that almost all human cancers differ in their karyotypic picture, and that the development of primary cancers in animals (either induced or spontaneous) is usually accompanied by diploidy [5, 22, 39, 54], even after metastases have developed, there are some recent findings bearing on this subject which are worthy of note:

A. A case of Burkitt's lymphoma has been described in which bilateral facial tumors and their regional metastases in the neck were shown to have different karyotypes [15]: one facial tumor and its metastases was diploid, whereas the others were definitely aneuploid. Unless one wishes to impute 2 different etiologic causes for the tumors, a most unlikely possibility, it would appear that the chromosomal changes do not play a part in the causation of Burkitt's lymphoma.

B. We have observed 2 cases, and others have also [16, 24], of acute myeloblastic leukemia in which the diploid picture observed at the initial phase of the disease changed to an aneuploid one during the course of the acute leukemia. Even though this is a very rare occurrence in acute myeloblastic leukemia, it does point to the evolution of karyotypic changes as secondary to the disease, rather than being the cause of it.

Much has been made of "marker" chromosomes as playing a primary role in human neoplasia [2, 10, 17, 28, 37, 57]. The occurrence of "markers" with allegedly distinct morphology in certain tumors is of interest, but lacks the consistency and specificity needed for reliable interpretation in relation to the primary causation of human cacer and leukemia. That "marker" chromosomes occur in human neoplasia is not surprising, particularly in view of what has already been discussed, i. e., that the human genome is a fragile thing and tends to rearrange and repair its chromosomes, often imperfectly, following induced damage. The evolution of "marker" chromosomes during the repair of the genome is a natural event, particularly since it is known that all kinds of structural abnormalities are present at all stages in the cells of human neoplastic tissues. It is possible that the genesis of "markers" may occur more frequently under some (e. g., solid tumor) and not under other conditions (e. g., chronic myelocytic leukemia or acute leukemia). Some tissues may be more susceptible to the emergence of one type of morphologic "marker" than another, e. g., C-Type chromosome in Burkitt's lymphoma [21, 23, 26, 61], large "markers" in paraproteinemia [14, 42, 59], double minutes [DMS] in neurogenic tumors [34, 51] (Fig. 4), etc. But, not all of these tumors, or for that matter not all the cells of any tumor, contain these "markers" and, furthermore, similar "markers" may be seen in tumors of different tissue origin. These statements do not detract from the significance of "marker" chromosomes in the progression and biologic behaviour of tumors, but they are intended to dampen the enthusiasm of those who think that "markers" are, in fact, directly involved in the genesis of human neoplasia.

A number of investigators has analyzed published data on the karyotypes of human cancer and leukemia (though some have utilized data not obtained in their own laboratories) and arrived at the conclusion that human neoplasia is characterized by a

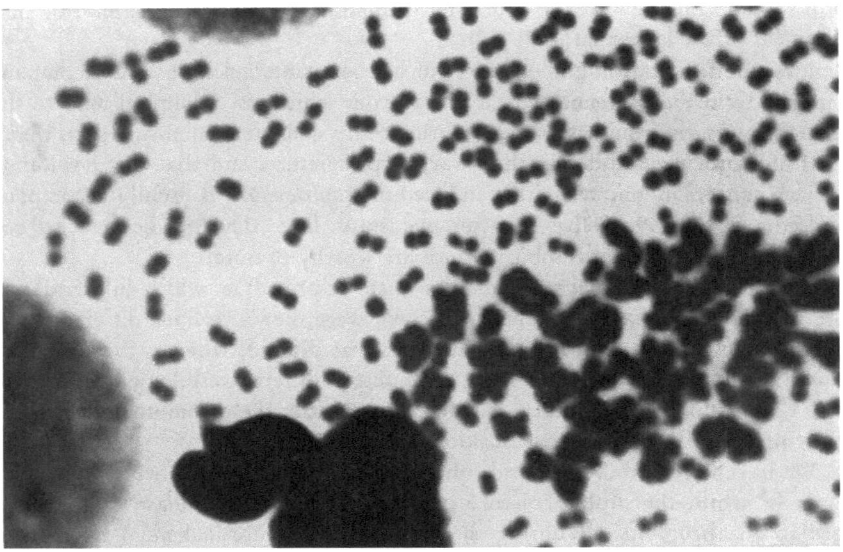

Fig. 4. Metaphase from the marrow of a patient with neuroblastoma. Note the presence of a large number of double minutes (DMS) chromosomes, probably resulting from the breakdown of some chromosomes in the cell

relative paucity of certain chromosomes [1, 27, 57], particularly in groups D, G and probably B, and by a relative excess of chromosomes in other groups (e. g., groups C and E), and that these changes may be causally related to human neoplasia. However, the chromosomes of groups D, G, and B are readily identified by the unique location of the centromere (acrocentric or near-telocentric) and, thus, can be readily classified morphologically. Even slight variations in the lengths of these chromosomes allow their exclusion from the normal set, due to the facile morphologic recognition of these aberrations. Furthermore, it is possible for "marker" chromosomes to be formed in such a way as to yield primarily metacentric or submetacentric units, which would then be included in the normal karyotypic groups (particularly C and E) due to the inability of the observers to recognize such abnormal "marker" chromosomes and differentiate them from those of the normal set. In addition, slight variations in the length of the metacentric or submetacentric chromosomes usually escape recognition and, hence, these chromosomes tend to be assigned to the normal chromosomal groups. The point being made here is that even if groups D, G, and B lack chromosomes in human cancers, and there is even disagreement with this concept also [47], the allegedly increased number of chromosomes in the other groups may be spurious due to the inability of the examiners to exclude these "abnormal" metacentric or submetacentric chromosomes from the normal groups. More importantly, since the overwhelming number of cancers is accompanied by one or more "markers", there is the distinct probability that autosomes of groups D, G and B may be more susceptible to "marker" formation and that this may account for the relative paucity of these chromosomes in human cancers.

In our laboratory a vectorial analysis of the karyotypes of human primary and metastatic cancers and *aneuploid* acute leukemias was performed to elucidate the evolution of chromosomal changes and their role in the genesis of neoplasia [47]. The analysis was based upon disagreements of the karyotypes of cancer and acute leukemic cells from the normal karyotypes and expressed as non-normality indices. The vectorial analysis took into account the karyotypes of *all* cells examined for each case and not a representative karyotype, as utilized by other investigators. Thus, it was shown that changes which occur in group C chromosomes are not due to fusion of autosomes from groups D and G. This contrast with the conclusion in other publications, in which only a karyotypic profile of each case was utilized, and stresses the need for more complete and comprehensive data on chromosomes in applying these to theories on the evolution of karyotypic changes in neoplasia. Cancers can be characterized often by a minimal vector, but this does not prove necessarily that "cloning" or that an evolutionary selection of one karyotype or another is an essential event in the *direct* genesis of cancer.

The remarkably variable cytogenetic picture that may be encoutered in early human neoplasia is a reflection of the lability and fragility of the human karyotype [1, 56], when affected by agents which lead to neoplasia. At this stage in the cancer development, it is still possible for the body to overcome the neoplastic process, even though karyotypic changes may be present. As the process becomes more stabilized and entrenched, however, selection of one karyotype over another occurs within the tumor, finally settling on one that endows it with more growth potential and advantages than afforded by other karyotypes. In the case of acute leukemia without chromosomal changes it is possible that cytogenetic abnormalities may be present in the initial stages of the disease but the cells with these karyotypic changes are eliminated, since the diploid set appears to be more favorable to the neoplastic process in these patients than afforded by aneuploid ones. The extreme rarity of diploid cancers may be related to the fact that such a genome does not favor local growth and metastatic spread of the cancer in human subjects. It has been shown upon careful analysis that in rat tumors with metastases, even though such metastatic lesions contained much of the basic karyotype of the primary tumor, they may further modify their chromosome constitution considerably [36]. Not only was diploidy present in the primary tumors, but it was also observed in the metastases of such tumors.

The sequence of cytogenetic events in human neoplasia would, thus, involve an initial direct or indirect (the latter as a result of metabolic alteration in the cell) insult on the genome, the insult also being the direct cause of the neoplasia, resulting possibly in the type of chromosomal changes observed in lymphocytes grown in culture and affected by noxious agents (chemicals, X-ray, viruses, etc.). Most of the cells with these changes, which consist of gaps, breaks, fragmentations, translocations, etc., are probably eliminated from the body. Only those cells survive which contain primarily a numerical change in chromosomal number due to faulty division and/or cells containing "marker" chromosomes due to recombination of parts of whole chromosomes due to the initial damage. With time, even though an array of cells with various karyotypes is available to the neoplastic process, it prefers to select one or another karyotype. Having said that the human genome is a fragile thing, why is it that generally the karyotypes of leukemic or cancer cells tend to remain rather stable throughout the course of the disease? An exception is the karyotypic change which occurs in the leukemic cells of patients with chronic myelocytic leukemia undergoing transformation to the blastic phase and the change from diploidy to aneuploidy in some cases of acute myeloblastic leukemia. It is possible that the neoplastic state endows the abnormal genome with resistance to change? Do further cytogenetic changes take place in neoplastic cells, but these are eliminated quickly and efficiently so that they are not discernable? Obviously, these questions will require more definite data before they can be answered.

We do not wish to imply that chromosomal aberrations may not play a part in tumor progression, once the neoplastic process is established. As a matter of fact, there are some indications that high ploidy in tumors favors metastases [1, 29, 31] and that shifts within the chromosome constitution of a cancer may occur with changes in the stage of the disease. However, these chromosomal changes always appear to be a variation on an already established karyotypic theme, with selection apparently favoring that cytogenetic profile which helps the cancer cells to survive. Attempts to correlate stage of malignancy, response to therapy, and other clinical and histological parameters with the karyotypic picture of tumors have been inconclusive, though much new data are necessary before this chapter can be considered closed. In previous publications we advanced the concept in the nature of a genetic oxymoron, that the karyotypic changes observed in the cells of human cancer and leukemia are, in fact, phenotypic expressions of the infinite variety in the genetic makeup of human subjects. As all of us differ in one respect or another (except for identical twins) in our genetic constitution, so does the karyotypic picture obtained in cancer and leukemia differ from one subject to another, as a result of the response and influence of the genome as reflected in the cytogenetic findings. The explanation just advanced does allow for similarity in cytogenetic changes in some individuals, but also explains the remarkable variations in the karyotypic changes observed in human neoplasia.

We do not insist on the hypothesis that chromosomal abnormalities are never involved in primary events of oncogenesis. There may be some neoplasms where such a causality exists, e. g., chronic myelocytic leukemia *and* the Ph^1-chromosome. However, based on our own experience and on the evidence available in the literature, we continue to believe that the chromosomal changes in most instances of neoplasia are epiphenomena. But we must emphasize that at the present time our efforts to elucidate the role of chromosomes in human neoplasia are restricted to the problem as to whether visible chromosomal abnormalities are present or not. A malignant cell with an apparent diploid chromosome constitution may well be characterized by profound structural changes in the chromosomes at the submicroscopic level and, certainly, by functional changes at the molecular level. Obviously, a modification or change in a single gene function would escape morphologic observation.

3. Possible Future Application of Cytogenetic Data in the Diagnosis and Treatment of Human Neoplasia

Even though much more data are needed, it is possible that cytogenetic findings in human cancer and leukemia may prove to be very valuable in the diagnosis and treatment of these diseases. More and more evidence is accumulating that invasion of a tumor and its response to therapy may be more directly related to its chromosome constitution, particularly if the number is near diploid, than to the histological picture. Furthermore, tumors with high ploidy (at least in cancer of the colon) tend to metastasize more readily than near-diploid ones [29]. Much remains to be done in evaluating the response of various cancers to X-ray or chemotherapy in relation to the cytogenetic picture of such tumors; and a correlation of the response of leukemias, particularly acute leukemias, to therapy of one type or another with the abnormal profile of the leukemia may prove to be of definite value in the treatment of these states. Are aneuploid leukemias more or less responsive to therapy than the diploid ones? Does hypodiploid acute myeloblastic leukemia differ in its clinical behavior from hyperdiploid acute myeloblastic leukemia? Only through an accumulation of a large body of cytogenetic data, conclusive and significant in every respect, will we be in a position to rely on such findings in the evaluation of chromosomal changes in the diagnosis, treatment and etiology of human neoplasia.

Conclusions

Even though we adhere to the view that microscopically visible chromosomal changes are not involved in the initial causation of human cancer and leukemia, we do not wish to detract from the real possibility of cytogenetic changes affording important leads and clues in the etiology, progression and treatment of these diseases. It is possible that the presence of double-minute (DMS) chromosomes in neurogenic tumors (Fig. 4), and occasionally in other types of cancers, may be indicative of the presence of a virus (oncogenic?) in such tumors. The genesis of certain characteristic "markers" in some tumors may yield a clue as to the possible etiology of the tumor. Furthermore, the biologic behavior of a tumor may be related to the presence of such "marker" chromosomes or to a unique aneuploidy, which may also play a role in the metastatic capability of the cancer. In fact, the presence of "marker" chromosomes of distinct morphology may possibly be related to the cause of the neoplasia and, thus, give us clues as to the possible etiology of the various human cancers.

Acknowledgements

The studies in our laboratory have been supported in part by a grant from the American Cancer Society, Inc., now VC-91L, formerly as T-182 and E-643K. I wish to thank Miss CHRISTINE HANSON for her clerical help. The author wishes to thank his many co-workers, who over the years have helped him in the study of chromosomal changes in human cancer and leukemia, but who are not responsible for and may, in fact, not agree with the views expressed in this paper. For these views the present author is solely responsible.

References

1. ATKIN, N. B.: In: Genetic Concepts and Neoplasia. Baltimore: The Williams and Wilkins, Co. 1970, p. 36.
2. ATKIN, N. B., BAKER, M. C.: J. nat. Cancer Inst. **36,** 539 (1966).
3. AUERSPERG, N., COREY, M. J., AUSTIN, G.: Lancet **1966 I,** 604.
4. ARRIGHI, F. E., HSU, T. C.: Cytogenetics **10,** 81 (1971).
5. BECKER, F. F., FOX, R. A., KLEIN, K. M., WOLMAN, S. R.: J. nat. Cancer Inst. **46,** 1261 (1971).
6. BERGER, R.: Ann. Génét. **8,** 70 (1965).
7. CASPERSSON, T., ZECH, L., JOHANSSON, C., MODEST, E. J.: Chromosoma **30,** 215 (1970).
8. CELLIER, K. M., KIRKLAND, J. A., STANLEY, M. A.: J. nat. Cancer Inst. **44,** 1221 (1970).
9. COX, D.: Brit. J. Cancer **22,** 402 (1968).
10. DEGROUCHY, J.: Ann. Génét. **9,** 55 (1966).
11. FORD, C. E., CLARKE, C. M.: Canad. Cancer Conf. **5,** 129 (1963).
12. FREED, J. J., SCHATZ, S. A.: Exp. Cell Res. **55,** 393 (1969).
13. GOFMAN, J. W., MINKLER, J. L., TANDY, R. K.: Clearing-house for Federal Scientific and Technical Information. National Bureau of Standards. Virginia: Springfield UCRL-50356, 1967.
14. GOH, K. O., SWISHER, S. N.: Amer. J. med. Sci. **260,** 237 (1970).
15. GRIPENBERG, U., LEVAN, A., CLIFFORD, P.: Int. J. Cancer **4,** 334 (1969).
16. GUNZ, F. W., RAVICH, R. B. M., VINCENT, P. C., STEWART, J. H., CROSSEN, P. E., MELLOR, J.: Ann. Génét. **13,** 79 (1970).
17. HAUSCHKA, T. A.: Cancer Res. **21,** 957 (1961).
18. HOSSFELD, D. K., SANDBERG, A. A.: Klin. Wschr. **48,** 1431 (1970).
19. HOSSFELD, D. K., HAN, T., HOLDSWORTH, R. N., SANDBERG, A. A.: Cancer (Philad.) **27,** 186 (1971).
20. HSU, T. C.: In: International Review of Cytology. Ed.: G. H. BOURNE and J. F. DANIELLI. New York and London: Academic Press 1961, pp. 69—161.
21. HUANG, C. C., MINOWADA, J., SMITH, R. T., OSUNKOYA, B. O.: J. nat. Cancer Inst. **45,** 815 (1970).
22. IKEUCHI, T., HONDA, T.: Cytologia (Tokyo) **36,** 173 (1971).
23. JACOBS, P. A., TOUGH, I. M., WRIGHT, D. H.: Lancet **1963 II,** 1143.
24. JENSEN, M. K.: Acta med. scand. **190,** 429 (1971).
25. KIRKLAND, J. A.: Obstet. gynec. Surv. **24,** 784 (1970).
26. KOHN, G., MELLMAN, W. J., MOORHEAD, P. S., LOFTUS, J., HENLE, G.: J. nat. Cancer Inst. **38,** 309 (1967).
27. LEVAN, A.: Hereditas (Lund) **55,** 28 (1966).

28. LEVAN, A., BIESELE, J. J.: Ann. N. Y. Acad. Sci. **71**, 1022 (1958).
29. LUBS, H. A.: In: Carcinoma of the Colon and Antecedent Epithelium. Ed.: W. J. BURDETTE. Springfield, Ill.: Charles C. Thomas 1970, pp. 319—332.
30. LUBS, H. A., SALMON, J. H.: J. Neurosurg. **22**, 160 (1965).
31. LUBS, H. A., KOTLER, S.: Ann. intern. Med. **67**, 328 (1967).
32. MAKINO, S.: Proc. intern. Genet. Symposia, Tokyo: 177, 1956, 1957.
33. MARK, J.: Europ. J. Cancer **6**, 489 (1970).
34. MARK, J., GRANBERG, I.: Acta neuropath. (Berl.) **16**, 194 (1970).
35. MINKLER, J. L., GOFMAN, J. W., TANDY, R. K.: Brit. J. Cancer **24**, 726 (1970).
36. MITELMAN, F., MARK, J.: Hereditas (Lund) **65**, 227 (1970).
37. MULDAL, S., ELEJALDE, R., HARVEY, P. W.: Nature (Lond.) **229**, 48 (1971).
38. NOWELL, P. C., HUNGERFORD, D. A.: J. nat. Cancer Inst. **25**, 85 (1960).
39. NOWELL, P. C., MORRIES, H. P., POTTER, V. R.: Cancer Res. **27**, 1565 (1967).
40. PARDUE, M. L., GALL, J. S.: Science **168**, **1356** (1970).
41. PROPP, S., LIZZI, F. A.: Blood **36**, 353 (1970).
42. ROCHON, M., CADOTTE, M., PRETTY, H. M., LONG, L. A.: L'Union Med. Canada **100**, 1750 (1971).
43. SANDBERG, A. A.: Cancer Res. **26**, 2064 (1966).
44. SANDBERG, A. A., AYA, T., IKEUCHI, T., WEINFELD, H.: J. nat. Cancer Inst. **45**, 615 (1970).
45. SANDBERG, A. A., CORTNER, J., TAKAGI, N., MAGHADAM, M. A., CROSSWHITE, L. H.: New Engl. J. Med. **275**, 809 (1966).
46. SANDBERG, A. A., TAKAGI, N., KATO, H.: In: The Proliferation and Spread of Neoplastic Cells. Baltimore: The Williams and Wilkins Co. 1968, pp. 99—136.
47. SANDBERG, A. A., BROSS, I. D. J., TAKAGI, N., SCHMIDT, M. L.: Cancer (Philad.) **21**, 77 (1968).
48. SANDBERG, A. A., TAKAGI, N., SUFONI, T., CROSSWHITE, L. H.: Cancer (Philad.) **22**, 1268 (1968).
49. SANDBERG, A. A., HOSSFELD, D. K.: Ann. Rev. Med. **21**, 379 (1970).
50. SANDBERG, A. A., HOSSFELD, D. K.: In: Cancer Medicine. Ed.: J. F. HOLLAND and E. FREI. Philadelphia, Pa.: Lea and Febiger 1972.
51. SANDBERG, A. A., SAKURAI, M., HOLDSWORTH, R. N.: Cancer (Philad.) **29**, 167 (1972).
52. SANDBERG, A. A., SAKURAI, M., FREEMAN, A. I., ELLISON, R. R.: 1972. Unpublished observations.
53. SANDBERG, A. A., HOSSFELD, D. K., EZDINLI, E. Z., CROSSWHITE, L. H.: Cancer (Philad.) **27**, 176 (1971).
54. SASAKI, M., MORI, M., KOBAYASHI, H., TAKEICHI, N.: Proc. Jap. Acad. **46**, 792 (1970).
55. SPIERS, A. S. D., BAIKIE, A. G.: Brit. J. Cancer **24**, 77 (1970).
56. SPRIGGS, A. I., BOWEY, C. E., COWDELL, R. H.: Cancer (Philad.) **27**, 1239 (1971).
57. STEENIS, H. V.: Nature (Lond.) **209**, 819 (1966).
58. TAKAGI, N., SANDBERG, A. A.: In: Axenic Mammalian Cell Reactions. Ed. G. L. TRITSCH, pp. 27—57.
59. TASSONI, E. M., DURANT, J. R., BECKER, S., KRAVITZ, B.: Cancer Res. **27**, 806 (1967).
60. TURPIN, R., LEJEUNE, J.: In: Les Chromosomes Humains. Paris: Gauthier-Villars 1965, pp. 181—215.
61. WHANG-PENG, J., GERBER, P., KNUTSEN, T.: J. nat. Cancer Inst. **45**, 831 (1970).
62. YAMADA, K., TAKAGI, N., SANDBERG, A. A.: Cancer (Philad.) **19**, 1879 (1966).
63. ZANKL, H., SINGER, H., ZANG, K. D.: Humangenetik **11**, 253 (1971).

Chromosome Alteration in the Course of Serial Transplantations of Experimental Tumors and Aging of Tumor Stemline Cells*

T. H. Yosida

According to our knowledge of cytogenetics, numerical and structural changes of chromosomes cause the change of genes or gene arrangements. Since the report of Boveri in 1912, many cytogeneticists have observed abnormal mitosis and the resultant chromosome changes in tumor cells and they have emphasized that the chromosome plays an important role in tumor development. In an early study of tumor cells, primary concern was directed to the abnormalities of cell division. Studies have been carried out on the solid tumors obtained from human patients and laboratory animals by use of the classical microtechnique.

The use of ascites tumor brought about great advances in this field of cytogenetics. Ascites rat tumor was first used by Makino and his school, and mouse ascites tumor mainly by Western scientists. On the basis of cytogenetical studies of Yoshida sarcoma, Makino in 1952 established a concept of tumor stemline in the transplantable tumors. According to him, a tumor has a cell lineage dividing regularly through cell generations with a characteristic chromosome constitution. Levan and Hauschka (1952) used a term "germ line" in almost the same context as "stemline". This concept of the stemline in transplantable tumors has been accepted by many cytogeneticists. The karyotype of the stemline, however, is not always constant but may change during serial transplantations under usual conditions.

1. Karyotype alterations in Yoshida rat sarcoma and MY mouse sarcoma. A typical case of the karyotype change during the course of tumor transfer was observed in the Yoshida rat sarcoma by Yosida 1959. In this case a few cells with a new marker chromosome (large J-shaped) developed in the course of serial transfers, and the number of mutated cells increased in parallel with the increase in number of the transfer generations. After the 20th transfer generation the cell population changed completely to a new stemline. In the MY mouse sarcoma was established by Yosida in 1960, the gross change of karyotype from diploidy to tetraploidy occurred after about the 90th transplant generation which corresponded to about 6 years. It is interesting that although the tumor with the diploid stemline could be transplanted successfully when it was in the diploid condition to only few mouse strains established in Japan, the tumor with tetraploid stemline could be trans-

---

* Contribution No. 889 from the National Institute of Genetics, Japan.

Supported by a grant-in-aid from the Ministry of Education of Japan (No. 92332).

Table 1. Change of transplantability in the MY mouse sarcoma in relation to ploidy shift of the tumor stem cells (Modified from YOSIDA *et al.*, 1960)

Strain of the mouse	Ploidy of tumor stem cells Diploidy		Tetraploidy	
SMA	62.2%[a]	(52)[b]	83.3%	(12)
SK	87.5	(16)	—	
S4	100.0	(62)	100.0	(19)
DM	76.5	(34)	18.0	(16)
D103	92.2	(51)	100.0	(30)
C3H	0	(70)	83.3	(12)
DBA	0	(6)	100.0	(17)
SWR	0	(11)	—	
Swiss albino	0	(8)	100.0	(12)
A	0	(10)	85.7	(14)
CBA	0	(3)	—	
C57BL	—		100.0	(11)
C58	—		94.1	(17)

[a] % of positive transplantation
[b] Number of mice used

planted to all mouse strains established in Japan and also to those imported from United States (Table 1).

2. Karyotype shift in mouse plasma cell tumors. Mouse plasma cell tumors, which are characterized generally by having a tetraploid karyotype, changed reapidly from diploidy to tetraploidy within one to two transplant generations (YOSIDA 1968; YOSIDA *et al.* 1968a, 1970). In this case it is interesting that when the karyotype of the tumor cell population changed from tetraploidy to hypotetraploidy, the cell line was able to continue to proliferate for a long time, but when it remained at the eutetraploid level the cells degenerated after a while, due to the depression of mitotic activity. Meanwhile, the diploid cells, which had been a minor component of the cell population, increased and overdominated the cell population again. In this diploid cell population, however, tetraploid cells again increased gradually, and the stemline eventually changed to tetraploid cells. A plasma cell neoplasm MSPC-1 established by us exhibited similar repeated tetraploidization during successive passages for about 2 years with a periodical cycle of several transfer generations. In order to determine whether the repeated ploidy alteration was accompanied by cell population changes, the karyotype was analysed in each diploid phase. Analysis of marker chromosomes appearing additively during serial passages showed that the cell population constituting one diploid phase was different from that of the next diploid phase, which was thus probably a variant of the former (MORIWAKI *et al.* 1971).

3. Karyotype shift in a rat chloroma (SHAY). Another interesting karyotype change was observed in the course of serial transplantations of the tumor cells of Shay's rat chloroma. According to NORWELL (1963) stemline cells of this tumor showed 43 chromosomes among which one extra chromosome in the group of medium sized acrocentrics (3—10) was observed. When the chromosome alignment was rearranged according to our system, one extra chromosome seems to be a trisomy of pair No. 3. During the 35th to 77th transplant generations in our laboratory the first

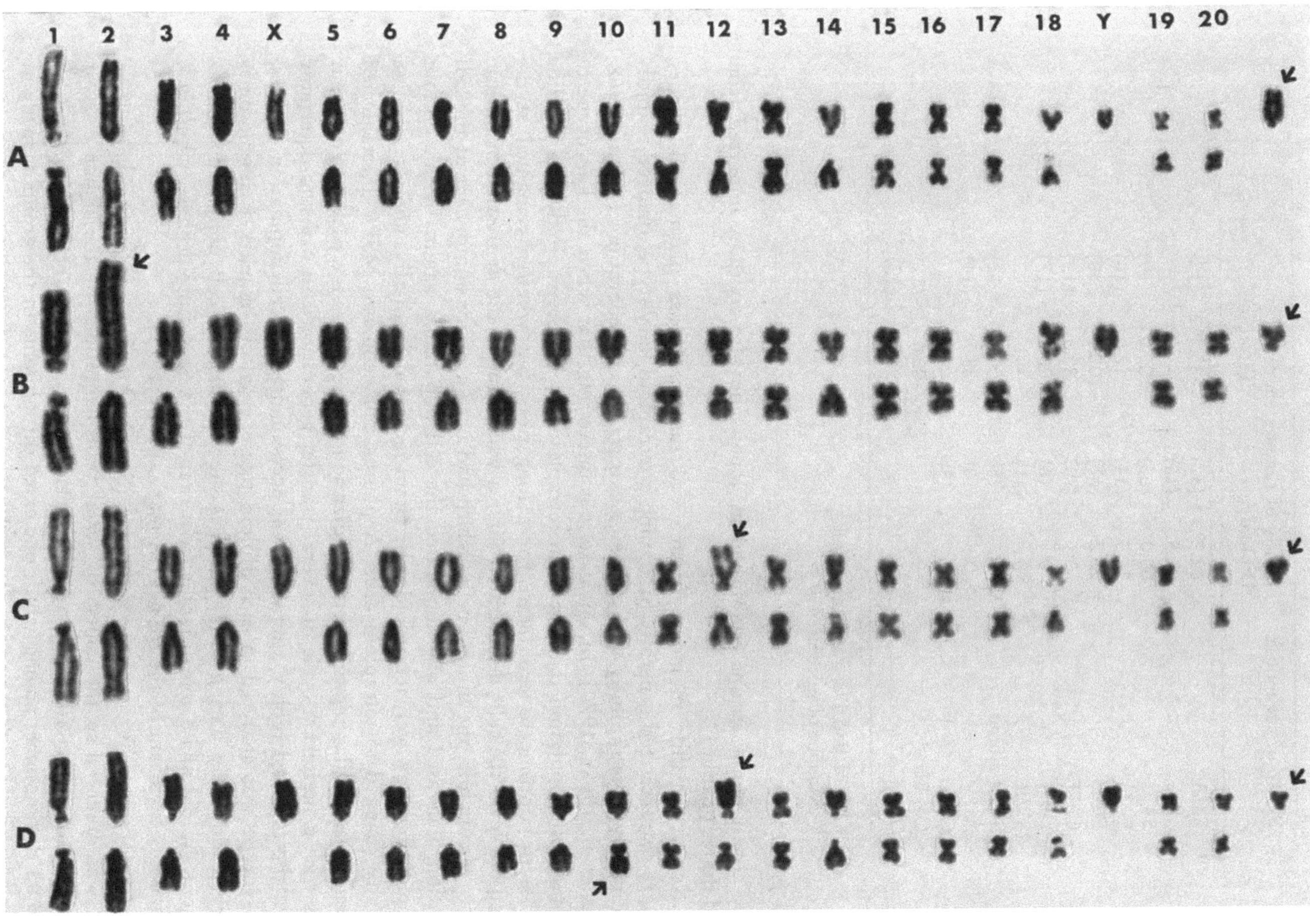

Fig. 1. Alteration of stemline karyotypes of a transplantable rat chloroma (SHAY) in the course of serial transplantations. A, from NORWELL (1963). B, in the 35th to 59 th transplant generations in Japan (1965—1967). C, in the 95th to 144th transplant generations in Japan (1968—1970). D, in the 179th transplant generation (1972). (Added new data to SAKAI, 1971)

chromosome alteration was observed. Namely, in the tumor stemline an extraordinary long acrocentric and a small subtelocentric chromosome were observed, whereas, the extra subtelocentric No. 3 detected by NORWELL was not found. Judging from the change in the markers it is suggested that breakage of the extra subtelocentric element occurred at the middle region of the long arm and the acentric chromosome segment was translocated to one of the No. 2 chromosomes, the other centric part remaining as the small subtelocentric marker (Fig. 1). (SAKAI *et al.* 1966, SAKAI 1971.)

At the 77th transplant generation a few cells with a large subtelocentric chromosome as a new marker were observed. In addidion to the appearance of the new marker, the extraordinarily large acrocentric chromosome was missing from the karyotype in the cells. Based on a comparative karyotype analysis of the original and the new mutant cells it was suggested that the acentric chromosome part which had been translocated to the No. 2 chromosome was retranslocated to one of the pair of No. 12 chromosomes. The frequency of cells with the new marker at the 77th transfer generation was only 5%, but at the 85th transfer generation it increased to 91%. At the 95th and 144th transfer generations all cells were found to have the new marker (Table 2). In the tumor cells at the 179th transplant generation (January, 1972), however, one submetacentric chromosome of medium size was observed for the first time, while one acrocentric chromosome of similar size was found to be missing from the stemline karyotype. It was assumed that one acrocentric chromosome, probably No. 11, in the preceding stemline cells underwent pericentric inversion resulting in the formation of the submetacentric chromosome. Fig. 2 shows the scheme of the sequential karyotype alteration in tumor cells of the rat chloroma (SHAY) in the course of serial transplantation. Chromosome alteration in this tumor occurred with a periodical cycle of about 2 or 3 years.

4. Ageing of tumor stemline cells. MAKINO (1952) emphasized that the most important of the tumor stemline was a constant of the stemline idiogram through many

Table 2. Karyotype alteration in the course of transfers of a rat chloroma (SHAY) (Added new data to SAKAI, 1971)

Years observed	Transpl. gener. in Japan	Chromosome number 37	40	41	42	43	44	45	46	No. of cells observed	% of cells with Karyotype[a] A	B	C
1965. 11 ∫ 1966. 1	35 ∫ 36	2	2	5	24	208	24	0	0	265	100	0	0
1966. 10 ∫ 1967. 2	52 ∫ 59				6	87	7			100	100	0	0
1967. 12	77					41	24	6	2	73	95	5	0
1968. 5	85				2	70	8	1	1	82	9	91	0
1968. 11	95			1	1	73	15	1		91	0	100	0
1969. 9	113			1	3	43	4			51	0	100	0
1970. 9	144				3	92	14	1		110	0	100	0
1972. 1	179		1	2	4	52	3			62	0	0	100

[a] Karyotype A: Cells with a long No. 2 acrocentric and an extra small subtelocentric markers. Karyotype B: Cells with a long No. 12 subtelocentric and an extraordinary subtelocentric markers. Karyotype C: Cells with type B markers and a submetacentric

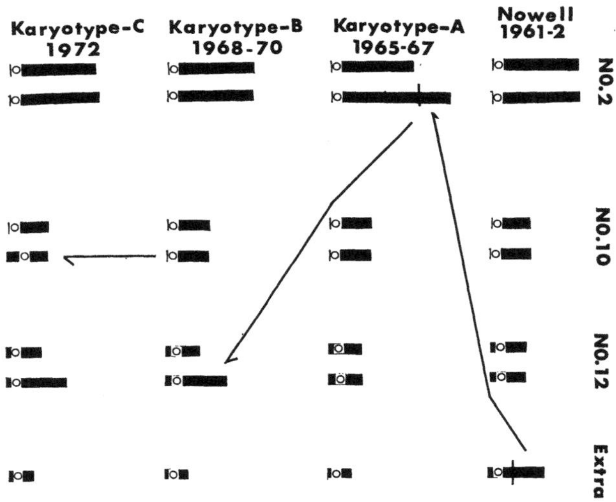

Fig. 2. Scheme of karyotype alterations of a rat chloroma (SHAY). (Added new data to SAKAI, 1971)

transfer generations. Later it was recognized that the stability of the stemline karyotype was not always absolute (MAKINO, 1957). Indeed the change in the tumor karyotype has been observed in the course of serial transplantations in several experimental tumors. HAUSCHKA and LEVAN (1958) emphasized that tumor progression was facilitated by continuous selective population shifts within a randomly mutating multiple stemline system. Based on the cytogenetical studies of several experimental tumors, it was explained (YOSIDA 1966b, 1968) that the karyotype alteration in the tumor stemline cells was dependent on sequential events of mutation and selection. Here it is necessary to consider the meaning of the constancy and the changeability of tumor stemline karyotype. If the gene or chromosomal mutations occurred frequently and continuously in tumor cells, a tumor stemline could not be established, because the tumor would then be composed of various mutant clones occurring in a random fashion. But many tumors show a modal distribution of chromosomes, which is refered to as the tumor stemline.

The problem remains why transplantable tumors have a stemline consisting of a certain karyotype through many generations, in spite of the continous and random occurrence of mutations in the cell population and whether this can be explained simply by sequential events of mutations and selection. In order to consolidate the different opinions on the behaviour of tumor stemline cells the idea of the "ageing" of the tumor cells is proposed (YOSIDA, 1972). All multicellular or unicellular organisms and sexually reproducing or asexually reproducing organisms exhibit the phenomenon of ageing. In the sexually reproducing organisms, the life can be extended by the recombination following the mating. Mating and recombination do not occur in the somatic cells, except the hybridization of *in vitro* cultured cells. In the normal human diploid cell strain, the diploid karyological character is limited to about 50 serial passages (or about one year) in *in vitro* culture as demonstrated by HAYFLICK and MOORHEAD (1961). Thereafter, mitotic activity decreases and aneuploidy appears (SAKSELA and MOORHEAD, 1963). Among the aneuploid cells a modal karyotype is observed as the stemline of the permanent cell line, but the stemline karyotype does not continue for many generations, before it is replaced by cells of another karyotype. In the human cell line, the life span of about 50 passages seems to reflect the ageing of the diploid cell strain. An aneuploid cell line arising after the diploid cell degeneration is the second stem cell population. The karyotype of the second stemline cells, however, is replaced by the tertiary stem cell population after a certain period by the mechanism described above. Thus, the proliferation of the re-established cell lines should be limited by "aging" as are the first diploid cells.

The karyotype alteration in the tumor stemline cells could be explained by the same mechanism. The only difference between the tumor strain and cultured lines is that the tumor strain growing *in vivo* will more strictly selected by immune responses than the cultured line growing *in vitro*. Therefore a karyotype of the tumor stemline may be stable as MAKINO demonstrated, but there is a limitation of the stability of the tumor stemline karyotype imposed by its age. Life span or age of the tumor stemline seems to be different for different strains of tumors (Fig. 3). Stemline A, which is characterized by a certain karyotype, degenerates after a certain transfer generations through ageing, and new cells with karyotype B, which occurred as a result of chromosomal alteration and selection from the stemline A increase in the cell population. Thus, the tumor is occupied by the new stemline B cells. The stemline B is eventually replaced by the stemline C by the same mechanism.

Why should the tumor stemline have a limited age and why do the tumor stemline cells degenerate after a certain period of cell multiplication? A possible explanation is that unfavourable genes may accumulate in the stemline cells during the progress of transplant generations. A chromosome alteration may be necessary to break the unfavourable function of the aged cells. A function change in cells following a ploidy shift or chromosome structural change in the tumor stemline has been demonstrated in many tumor strains. A change in enzyme activity after a ploidy change was demonstrated in Ehrlich ascites tumor by KID and GROSS (1959),

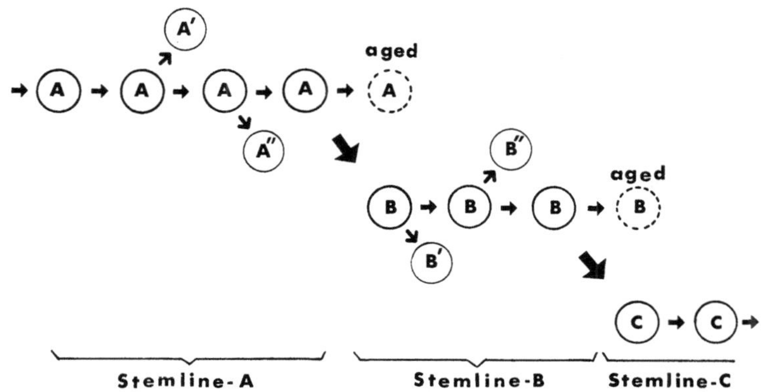

Fig. 3. Mode of alteration of stemline karyotype in the course of tumor transplantations by ageing of tumor stemline cells. A, B and C are stemline cells. A′, A″, B′ and B″ are mutant cells which could not develop as new stemline cells. Degeneration of the cell is shown by the broken circle

TSUKADA and FU (1959), and in cultured hepatic cells by KONIGSBERG and NITOWSKY (1962). Quantitative changes in protein synthesis following a karyotype shift has been demonstrated in the Yoshida sarcoma and mouse plasma cell tumors (MORIWAKI *et al.*, 1969). The change in the ability to infiltrate into organs, which has been demonstrated in the karyological mutants of the Yoshida rat sarcoma and Ehrlich mouse tumor (YOSIDA, 1959, 1964) may be due to the change of cell surface antigens as considered by HAUSCHKA *et al.* (1956), SACKS and GALLILY (1956) and AMOS (1956).

Does the functional change of tumor cells brought about by the chromosome alteration reflect the rejuvenation of cell lineage? Unfavourable genes accumulated in the cell would not be detrimental to the mutated cells which may have functions differing from the parent one. The gross change of stemline karyotype has been demonstrated in the resistant cell lines which developed after repetitive treatment with some chemicals (YOSIDA, 1966 a; YOSIDA *et al.*, 1967, 1968 b). Mutant cell lines thus established were not only resistant to the chemicals, but sometimes required such chemicals to maintain cell life and were thus described as a dependent mutant line (POTTER and LAW, 1957). In the light of these observations, it can be said that the change in gene function following the chromosomal alteration might play an important role in the rejuvenation of the aged stemline cells. Thus, the tumor stemline evolves by karyotype alteration and the transplantable tumor continues its life through many cell generations.

Summary

Karyotype alterations in tumor stemline cells are to be seen during tumor transfers (increasing with the numbers of transplant generations). This is an effect of "aging" of the tumor cells.

References

AMOS, D. B.: Ann. N. Y. Acad. Sci. **63**, 706 (1956).
BOVERI, T.: Frage der Entwicklung maligner Tumoren. Jena 1912.
HAUSCHKA, T. S.: Trans. N. Y. Acad. Sci. Ser. II. **16**, 64 (1953).
HAUSCHKA, T. S., KVEDAR, B. J., GRINELL, S. T. *et al.*: Ann. N. Y. Acad. Sci. **63**, 683 (1956).
HAUSCHKA, T. S., LEVAN, A.: J. nat. Cancer Inst. **21**, 77 (1958).
HAYFLICK, L., MOORHEAD, P. S.: Exp. Cell Res. **25**, 585 (1961).
KID, S., GROSS, A. L.: Biochim. biophys. Acta (Amst.) **36**, 185 (1959).
KONIGSBERG, U. R., NITOWSKY, H. M.: J. nat. Cancer Inst. **29**, 699 (1962).
LEVAN, A., HAUSCHKA, T. S.: Hereditas (Lund) **38**, 251 (1952).
MAKINO, S.: Chromosoma (Berl.) **4**, 649 (1952).
MAKINO, S.: Int. Rev. Cytol. **6**, 26 (1957).
MORIWAKI, K., IMAI, H. T., YOSIDA, T. H.: Jap. J. Genet. 44, Suppl. **2**, 71 (1969).
MORIWAKI, K., IMAI, H. T., YAMASHITA, J., YOSIDA, T. H.: J. nat. Cancer Inst. **47**, 623 (1971).
NOWELL, P. C., FERRY, S., HUNGERFORD, A.: J. nat. Cancer Inst. **30**, 687 (1963).
POTTER, M., LAW, L. W.: J. nat. Cancer Inst. **18**, 413 (1956).
SACKS, L., GALLILY, R.: J. nat. Cancer Inst. **16**, 803 (1956).
SAKAI, T.: Acta Heam. Jap. **34**, 604 (1971).
SAKAI, T., YOSIDA, T. H., SHIMIZU, M.: Ann. Rep. nat. Inst. Genet. Jap. **16**, 51 (1966).
SAKSELA, E., MOORHEAD, P. S.: Proc. nat. Acad. Sci. (Wash.) **50**, 390 (1963).

TSUKADA, H., FU, S. C. J.: Proc. Amer. Ass. Cancer Res. **3**, 70 (1959).
YOSIDA, T. H.: Z. Krebsforsch. **63**, 209 (1959).
YOSIDA, T. H.: Gann **50**, 233 (1959).
YOSIDA, T. H.: Jap. J. Genet. **38**, 342 (1964).
YOSIDA, T. H.: Jap. J. Genet. **41**, 59 (1966 a).
YOSIDA, T. H.: Jap. J. Genet. **41**, 439 (1966 b).
YOSIDA, T. H.: Cancer Cell in Culture. Ed. H. KATSUTA. Tokyo: Univ. Tokyo Press 1968, p. 171.
YOSIDA, T. H.: Proc. Jap. Acad. **48**, 268 (1972).
YOSIDA, T. H., ISHIHARA, T., HAMADA, T.: Gann **51**, 55 (1960).
YOSIDA, T. H., OHARA, K., LAW, L. W.: Jap. J. Genet. **42**, 338 (1967).
YOSIDA, T. H., IMAI, H. T., POTTER, M.: J. nat. Cancer Inst. **41**, 1083 (1968 a).
YOSIDA, T. H., OHARA, H., ROOSA, R. A.: Jap. J. Genet. **43**, 49 (1968 b).
YOSIDA, T. H., IMAI, H. T., MORIWAKI, K.: J. nat. Cancer Inst. **45**, 411 (1970).

Early Changes in Ploidy and Cytogenetics of Liver Cells After Diethylnitrosamine Treatment

H. WRBA, P. FISCHER, M. WEISSBERG, and L. WIEST

Changes in function and growth in the liver cell can be produced by relatively simple experimental mechanisms. All types of growth-changes, embryonic, regenerative and malignant are easy to induce.

We have been engaged for a considerable time in the study of tumor growth regulation in this organ through the determination of protein and DNA synthesis (WRBA and RABES, 1967). By using a type of *in vitro* confrontation technique, viz. explanation of organs in a system in which only a humoral exchange through the media is possible, we have been able to demonstrate the induction of many regulatory precursors — for example in the resumption of respiration in explanted cells of normal adult liver confronted with regenerating liver (RABES and WRBA, 1965). Such experiments have demonstrated the presence of "regeneration factors" in the regenerating liver. These findings have been recently confirmed (LEFFERT *et al.*, 1972).

The liver of all newborn mammals is composed entirely of diploid cells. In the course of further development, ploidy increases. In the mouse and rat, the number of diploid cells falls progressively after birth as shown in Fig. 1. The number of binucleate cells increases to a level of about 30%. In the mature animal approxi-

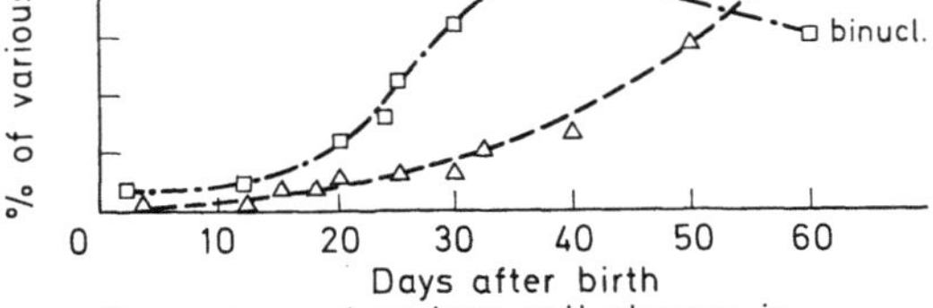

Percentage of various cell classes in the liver parenchyma of rats mately 70% of cells are tetraploid, while somewhat less than 10% of all liver cells are normally octoploid. In man, this alteration in liver ploidy begins at puberty.

After excision of the pituitary in rats, the percentage of tetraploid cells falls from 70 to 20% in 70 days. This continuous fall is associated with a simultaneous increase in the number of diploid cells. The number of polyploid cells also decreases (WIEST, 1969).

After partial hepatectomy the number of polyploid cells increases rapidly. Twenty-four hours after the removal of the suprarenals, the number of polyploid cells in the liver lies between 70 and 80%. The mitotic rate also rises after hepatectomy and to a moderate degree after adrenalectomy. DNA synthesis 24 hours after hepatectomy is increased several times over the control rate. After adrenalectomy the rise is only on third of the post-hepatectomy rate.

In general one can state that increases in DNA synthesis and in ploidy development run parallel, while a decrease or suppression of DNA synthesis in the liver after hypophysectomy is also correlated with a fall in ploidy.

The determination of liver ploidy was arrived at in each case by two independent methods — by cytophotometry in histological sections, and by measurement of isolated liver cells from dissociated liver tissue. The dissociation and evaluation of isolated liver cells is essential for identification of binucleate cells (WIEST, 1969).

We also investigated the effect of the liver specific diethylnitrosamine (DENA) on liver ploidy and DNA synthesis. Newborn animals were chosen after consideration of the perinatal action of the drug and the similarity in ploidy of all liver cells in the newborn. After only one application of 10 mg DENA/kg on the day of birth a marked and unexpected result was obtained. After 24 hours there was a significant rise in the number of tetraploid cells which was maintained until the appearance of microcarcinomas on the 30th day. Animals from the same litter were used as controls (WIEST, 1972).

The action of this carcinogenic drug as early as 24 hours after a single application was a reproducible finding. This early significant change seems to us to be of importance — almost immediately after the application of DENA, tetraploid cells appear. During the course of the experiment it is possible to follow the appearance after 10 days of 8n, after 25 days of 16n, and later of very high ploidy cells. It is noteworthy that during this development, binucleate cells, which in the untreated animal increase visibly from the 10th day onwards, are practically non-existent in the DENA treated animal. It is known from the literature that the increase of polyploid cells in the normal liver occurs through an intermediary stage, namely the production of binucleate diploid cells. In contrast, in the liver of DENA treated newborn rats, a logarithmic decrease of ploidy is to be seen. This apparently meaningful suppression of binucleate cells by this liver specific carcinogen is strictly dose dependent.

Newborn rats, treated with different doses of DENA (0.1; 0.2; 0.4; 0.5; 1.0 and 10 mg DENA/kg body weight) demonstrate a definite dose-dependent fall in binucleate cells in the liver from 40% to between 2—4% (Fig. 2). In adult animals, an increase in high ploidy cells is apparent within 24—72 hours after hepatectomy. According to investigations of GRUNDMANN (GRUNDMANN, 1967), the administration of DENA causes a decrease in polyploidy, which was the beginning of the malignant growth. In the DENA damaged liver (16 mg DENA/kg for 3 weeks) we

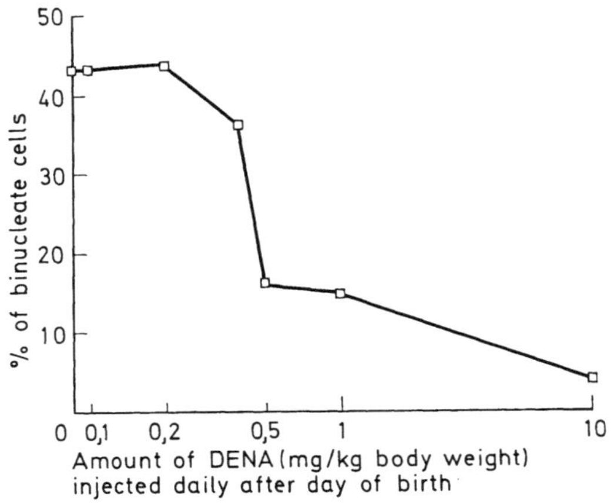

have found an increase in DNA synthesis compared with the norm, which was, however, a suppression compared with the partially hepatectomised animal (MOHR *et al.,* 1968). In the normal newborn rat DENA causes absolutely no suppression of DNA synthesis but is apparently effective in preventing the amitotic division of binucleate cells.

An equally characteristic change in the liver cells of newborn rats has been demonstrated by cytogenetic analysis. Little has as yet been published on the early cytogenetic effects of chemical carcinogens. We have undertaken a systematic cytogenetic analysis of liver and spleen of newborn Sprague Dawley rats after administration of DENA. In each experiment one litter of approximately 8 animals was used. Half the animals received a daily dose of 10 mg DENA/kg by subcutaneous injection in the 1st, 2nd, 3rd, 7th, 10th and 12th day after birth and subsequently at intervals of approximately 10 days, until the appearance of carcinomas. The application of DENA produced no change in the first and second day in comparison with controls. From the 3rd day, however, about 50% of the metaphases examined showed losses in the region of the small metacentric chromosomes. Chromosomes nos. A7 or B5, and sometimes both, were often monosomic or completely absent. These changes persisted until the histological appearance of hepato-cellular carcinomas. Metaphases from spleens and bone marrows of these animals remained normal throughout (GROVER and FISCHER, 1971).

Summary

Liver ploidy was measured by cytophotometry in histological sections and after isolation of liver cells. Diethylnitrosamine increased the DNA synthesis of the liver cells and prevented the amitotic division of binucleate cells. The same carcinogen produced deletions of the chromosomes A7 and/or B5 when injected subcutanously into newborn rats beginning on the 3rd day after birth.

References

GROVER, S., FISCHER, P.: Europ. J. Cancer 7, 77 (1971).

GRUNDMANN, E.: In: Control of Cellular Growth in Adult Organisms. Eds. H. TEIR and T. RYTÖMAA. London and New York: Academic Press 1967.

MOHR, U., SPEETZEN, R., KNECHT, M., WRBA, H.: Z. Naturforsch. **23 b/4**, 528 (1968).

LEFFERT, H., PAUL, D., SATO, G., HOLLEY, R. W.: Proc. nat. Acad. Sci. (Wash.) **69**, 374 (1972).

RABES, H., WRBA, H.: Exp. Cell Res. **39**, 669 (1965).

WIEST, L.: Verh. dtsch. path. Ges., 53. Tagg., Stuttgart: Gustav Fischer 1969.

WIEST, L.: Mikroskopie **25**, 401 (1969).

WIEST, L.: Europ. J. Cancer (in press, 1972).

WRBA, H., RABES, H.: Control of Cellular Growth in Adult Organisms. Eds. H. TEIR and T. RYTÖMAA. London and New York: Academic Press 1967.

Carcinogenesis *in vitro*

J. Pontén

Studies *in vitro* of oncogenic agents have attained an ever increasing importance mainly because of the precision and ease by which events at the cellular and subcellular level can be followed. This article will examine the relevance of such data for the understanding of a much more complicated process — the development of spontaneous malignant tumors *in vivo*. This seems particularly important in view of the enormous current interest in the possibility that human cancers may be caused by RNA viruses — a hypothesis largely resting on observations *in vitro*.

A special terminology has grown up for cells in culture. They are said to be transformed when they show certain permanent abnormalities. Three operationally distinct forms of transformations have been defined (Table 1).

Table 1. Characteristics of three operationally defined types of cell transformation *in vitro*

Type of alteration	Synonyms	Essential features
irregular growth transformation	lack of the contact inhibition of locomotion	failure of intercellular contact to paralyze cell membrane motion (persisting activity of lamellipodia)
unrestrained growth transformation	lack of the density dependent inhibition of cell multiplication	persisting cell proliferation in densely concentrated cell populations (increased terminal cell density)
infinite growth transformation	establishment of a permanent cell line	capacity of cells to undergo an infinite number of divisions

Implicit in Table 1 is the understanding that normal cells do not show any of the listed transformations. This has been amply demonstrated for fibroblasts and later for glia and other cells, the growth of which is normally subject to stringent regulation *in vitro*. Cell locomotion, which is principally carried out by a special organ, i. e. the leading edge with its lamellipodia, is checked in fibroblasts, glia and epithelia by contact with other cells so that they adhere to each other along immobilized segments of their respective membranes. Locomotion becomes restricted by this mechanism and dense cell populations will form a tissue-like structure where immobile cells are held in fixed positions. The mechanism by which membranes are paralyzed and made to adhere to each other is unknown.

Cell proliferation is likewise normally under strict control. As cell density increases and confluency is reached, the multiplication rate drops rapidly until it becomes virtually zero. Cells are then said to be resting at their terminal density which is expressed as number of cells per unit growth area. The mechanism is unknown but cannot be explained on the basis of exhaustion of the medium or its constituent growth factors. Instead special intercellular relations are created (topoinhibition) which either trigger inhibitory or suppress stimulatory signals at the cell periphery, which determine whether or not the cell is to enter the growth cycle.

Table 2. Type of fibroblast or glia transformation

Procedure	Abnorm. membr. motility (irregular growth)		Uncontrolled DNA synth. (unrestrained growth)		Infinite multiplication (infinite growth)	
	unstable species (mouse etc.)	stable species (man, chicken etc.)	unstable species (mouse etc.)	stable species (man, chicken etc.)	unstable species (mouse etc.)	stable species (man, chicken etc.)
serial cultivation	– or +	–	– or +	–	+	–
chemical carcinog.	+	–[a]	+	–[a]	+	–[a]
oncog. DNA virus	– or +[a]	– or +[a]	+	+	+	– (or +)[b]
oncog. RNA virus	+	+	+	+	+	–
explanted cancer	+	+	+	+	+	+

[a] no extensive data exist
[b] refers to occasional human lines

The third type of control is one of the great mysteries of cell biology. Its effect is to prevent normal fibroblasts, glia and epithelia from undergoing an infinite number of divisions. Fibroblasts and glia may for instance go through 20 or more cell cycles in perfect condition only to enter a declining stage (phase III) which eventually terminates in cell extinction. The invariable deterioration of normal cells in culture is not due to exhaustion of nutrients. It has speculatively been called ageing at the cellular level. Again the mechanism for "cellular ageing" is unknown.

Many agents have been shown to induce the alterations listed in Table 1. With few exceptions the same agents are also oncogenic *in vivo*, while factors incapable of transforming cells *in vitro* do not induce cancer in animals either. This close parallelism has naturally led people to believe that transformation *in vitro* is the same process as carcinogenesis *in vivo*. Careful analysis will, however, show that such a statement needs qualification.

Fibroblasts and glia cells are two well defined species of cells capable of serial passage in culture. Table 2 summarizes several important facts about transformation of these cells *in vitro*. It is seen that serial cultivation *per se* causes infinite growth transformation in certain species which are described as unstable. The best example of an unstable species is the mouse, but spontaneous infinite growth transformation is also frequent among rat and hamster fibroblasts. Stable species, in contrast, do not give rise to lines with a capacity for endless multiplication. Human and chicken cells are well known examples.

Lines which have undergone spontaneous infinite growth transformation usually also show a disturbed control of membrane motility and density-dependent DNA synthesis. It is, however, possible to isolate lines which, in spite of infinite growth transformation, retain an apparently normal control of cell locomotion and division. The 3T3 mouse line of Todaro is the prime example.

Infinite growth transformation is closely correlated with tumorigenicity *in vivo*. In all well controlled studies syngeneic cells have given rise to tumors upon implantation with the possible exception of 3T3-like variants.

The species-determined instability constitutes a serious experimental difficulty in the evaluation of the effects of applied carcinogens. As chemical carcinogens have not been shown to transform stable cells it is not known if their transforming ability in unstable systems is an enhancement of an inherent tendency or a genuine effect on the target cell.

The oncogenic DNA viruses cause infinite growth transformation in stable species only with difficulty, at least if one generalizes from the only thoroughly investigated system (SV40/human fibroblasts). Their main effect is to disturb density-controlled initiation of the cell cycle. After transformation by SV40, the local density at which inhibition of cell multiplication is first seen may be increased by a factor of 5 or more. The effect on membrane motility has never been extensively investigated with sophisticated techniques (time-lapse filming, scanning EM), but indirect evidence suggests that the membrane function is altered, for instances in polyoma virus transformed hamster cells which acquire the capacity to grow in soft agar.

The oncogenic RNA viruses exert their main effect on the cell membrane motility. The membrane becomes hyperexcitable, partially uninhibitable by contact with other cells and the site of "atypical ruffling", i. e. formation of lamellipodia at points where ruffling is never normally seen. The effect is an abnormal locomotion which, for instance, may give the cells the capacity to traverse each other. The membrane alteration is intimately coupled with characteristic cytological changes which can be distinguished from all other morphological alterations induced *in vitro*. The other main but less consistent effect is a reduced density-dependent inhibition of cell proliferation. Oncogenic RNA viruses may prolong the life span of transformed cultures but have never been shown to have the capacity to cause infinite growth transformation in two well investigated stable species (human, chicken).

Cells transformed *in vitro* should be compared with cells from cancers already established *in vivo*. When unstable species are considered no principal differences emerge. However, if stable species are considered (man and chicken are the only well studied examples) the picture is not so clear, as differences in behaviour are apparent between man and chicken, which are the only well studied examples.

Chicken sarcomas induced by inoculation of RNA viruses behave identically to fibroblasts transformed by the same agents *in vitro*. The morphology is highly characteristic and, in spite of a profound disturbance in cellular motility and density-dependent proliferation control, infinite growth transformation is not present. The cells die out when carried *in vitro* or *in vivo*. One exception is lymphosarcoma induced by lymphomatosis virus. About 50% of these tumors become serially transplantable *in vivo*.

Spontaneous tumors of a stable species have been difficult to study *in vitro*. Only recently has it become possible to cultivate a reasonable proportion of human cancers. In our laboratory 15 glioma and 3 sarcoma lines have been extensively studied and in all of them irregular and/or unrestrained growth transformation could be established in addition to the infinite growth transformation. We can therefore conclude that human cancer lines from spontaneous neoplasms which can be grown successfully *in vitro* have a more extensive break-down of normal controls than human lines transformed by carcinogens *in vitro*.

Speculations about the significance of *in vitro* cell transformation for the understanding of spontaneous cancers can be divided into two categories.

One outlook is that cell transformation *in vitro* is an entirely irrelevant system. It does not reveal the same features as those found in natural tumors. Of the two stable species so far well studied only in the chicken is there a correspondence between the effect of a natural carcinogen (RNA viruses) *in vivo* and *in vitro*. In man, normal cells are susceptible to viral transformation but the resulting cell populations clearly deviate from those derived from spontaneous tumors. One might, therefore, believe that those factors which are efficient *in vitro* may not be the natural carcinogens. This could be particularly damaging for the theory that RNA viruses cause sarcomas and leukemias in man. It is highly desirable to continue work on human neoplasms *in vitro* to settle this question.

A second, more productive, attitude asserts that transformation *in vitro*, particularly of stable cells without the disturbing background tendency of spontaneous transformation, gives a profound insight into phenomena of fundamental interest in tumor biology. Viruses and carcinogens effective *in vitro* should be looked upon as valuable experimental tools rather than putative natural human carcinogens. From this point of view it has become clear that human fibroblasts and glia are acted upon by DNA and RNA viruses in the same way as are cells of other vertebrates.

We have made some preliminary comparisons between spontaneous gliomas and glia cells transformed by feline sarcoma virus (FSV) and SV40 as examples of RNA and DNA tumor viruses. The overall general impression is that both viruses cause a much more pronounced irregular and unrestrained growth transformation than that found in the spontaneously induced tumor cells but that it is at least operationally quantitatively similar. It therefore seems logical to assume that these viruses only turn on certain defined partial expressions of the neoplastic state but that they cannot induce the entire spectrum of changes which underlies carcinogenesis in man.

The reason for this failure may be trivial. It is possible that selection and other factors *in vivo* so modify the response to a carcinogen that superimposed alterations mask the viral-dependent traits. It is, however, equally likely that carcinogenesis *in vivo* is a multifactorial process in contrast to transformation *in vitro* which is induced by only one factor. It would be of great value to find out how normal stable cells respond to a combination of carcinogens such as hydrocarbons plus an RNA virus. Will we then see a response which is more like that seen *in vivo*?

Summary

Many agents are able to induce *in vitro* the three types of cell transformation defined as: 1. Lack of contact inhibition of locomotion, 2. Lack of density dependent inhibition of cell multiplication and 3. Establishment of a permanent cell line. Differences between carcinogenesis *in vitro* and *in vivo* are apparent, but the effects of viruses and carcinogens *in vitro* can be regarded as valuable experimental tools. Feline sarcoma virus (FSV) and SV40, examples of RNA and DNA tumor viruses, cause in glia cells a much more pronounced irregular and unrestrained growth transformation than that found in the spontaneously induced glioma cells. The reason for this difference is unknown and has to be the aim of further investigations.

Induction and Some Characteristics of "Minimal Deviation" and Other Transplantable Rat Hepatomas

H. P. MORRIS and D. R. MERANZE

During the last two decades we have induced a large number of hepatomas and other types of tumors in inbred strains of rats at sites distant from the site of administration. The chemical carcinogens used have been incorporated at different dosage levels into adequate diets of natural food stuffs. Many of the primary hepatomas have been transplanted to new hosts of the strain of origin. Most, but not all, of these primary tumors grew in the new hosts. The tumors that grew have been maintained by serial transfer. These transplantable tumors are characterized by different rates of growth as measured by time between transfers. The size of the tumors at time of transfer is also highly correlated with growth rate.

These transplanted tumors provide a spectrum of experimental tumor models that differ by 20-fold or more in growth rate. They are invaluable for investigators to use to study the biological and biochemical parameters associated with different degrees of malignancy and to better define the essential from the non-essential alterations that upset the normal regulatory mechanisms in homeostasis.

This hepatoma spectrum has been arranged in Table 1 of pages with the slowest growing tumor appearing first and, the fastest growing tumor last. Growth rate was measured by months between transfers. The slowest growing tumor we now have averages 12.5 months between transfers. While the most rapid growing tumor averages 0.6 months between transfers. The slow growing tumors are well- to highly-differentiated. The fast growing tumors are poorly-differentiated. The intermediate growth rate tumors are usually well-differentiated to a mixture either of well- to poorly- or well- to highly-differentiated cells. Several tumors have the diploid number of chromosomes but only three of all we have induced have a normal karyotype.

Tumors having a transfer time averaging 1.2 months or less were usually poorly-differentiated. Those tumors having transfer times of 1.5 months to 12.5 months were well- to highly-differentiated with only a few overlaps.

The same data arranged according to the inducing agent is shown in the Table 2 on pages 105/106. Several different levels of feeding the carcinogen, FdiAA, are shown on the first two pages. No well-differentiated tumors were induced at 1.8 mM/kg of diet. Several diploid tumors were induced at a feeding level of 0.56 mM/kg of diet but no diploid tumors were found in a repeat experiment at the same level of feeding.

Each of the three diploid tumors with a normal karyotype was induced by a different chemical carcinogen. It is our experience that a high level of a very active

Table 1. Transplantable hepatomas histo and biological characteristics (Cont'd)

Tumors	Inducing agent	Level mM/kg	Generations used	Months between transfers Avg.	Histological type	Metastases −/+	Chromosome number	Primary sex
20	10	0.005	1—3	12.6	HD-WD	3/0	—	M
66	9	1.12	1—2	11.5	HD	2/0	42 NK	M
21	10	0.005	1—4	10.8	HD	3/0	—	M
16	10	0.005	1—4	10.5	W-WD	3/0	42—44	M
9618B	3	1.13	1—2	10.0	W-HD	4/0	42—44	M
9618A	3	1.13	1—5	8.0	HD	14/1	42 NK	M
47C	1	0.56	1—4	7.7	HD	1/3	—	M
39A	1	0.56	1—5	7.2	HD-WD	2/4	—	M
7787	2	1.27	7—14	6.3	HD-WD	8/0	44	F
28A	1	0.56	2—5	6.0	HD	2/2	82—85	M
44	1	0.56	1—4	5.8	WD	3/1	85	M
6	10	0.005	1—5	5.5	HD-WD	5/0	—	M
8624 [a]	4	1.12	12	4.7	WD-HD	—	—	M
42A	1	0.56	1—4	4.7	WD	3/1	—	M
9633	6	0.88	1—10	4.0	WD	3/2	42 NK	M
R3B	1	0.94	3—15	4.1	WD	5/5	43	M
9633F	6	0.88	5—9	4.0	WD	2/2	—	M
7794B	2	1.27	10—17	3.1	HD	2/8	44	M
7794A	2	1.27	23—30	2.9	WD	6/1	42	M
R7	1	0.94	4—19	2.8	WD	4/6	44	M
38B	1	0.56	2—12	2.5	WD	8/2	—	M
9611B	3	1.13	10—16	2.5	HD-WD	2/5	42—43	M
38A	1	0.56	1—2	2.3	WD	2/0	—	M
8995	8	1.10	18—26	2.3	WD	0/10	43	M
9108	1	0.56	20—29	2.0	WD	4/6	42	M
5123C	2	1.27	71—77	2.0	WD	2/8	96	F
7793	2	1.27	21—28	1.8	WD	2/8	45	F
8994	8	1.10	29—38	1.8	Pd	9/1	72—82	M
7316B	7	1.11	32—41	1.8	WD	4/6	55	F
7795	2	1.27	29—39	1.8	WD	1/8	46—47	M
7800	2	1.27	42—48	1.7	WD	2/8	42	M
H35	1	0.94	55—64	1.7	WD	5/5	43—44	M
9121F	1	0.56	20—29	1.7	WD	8/2	—	M
7316A	7	1.11	33—42	1.6	WD	0/10	43	F
R1	1	0.94	22—31	1.6	WD	1/9	46	M
5123D	2	1.27	70—80	1.6	WD-Pd	0/10	45	F
5123A	2	1.27	80—89	1.5	WD	0/10	46	F
9121	1	0.56	24—33	1.5	WD	10/0	42	M
5123B	2	1.27	93—102	1.2	WD-Pd	4/6	46	F
$9618A_2$	3	1.13	4—13	1.2	Pd	6/4	41	M
9098	1	0.56	32—41	1.2	WD-HD	7/3	42	M
5123tc	2	1.27	78—86	1.2	WD-Pd	1/9	47—49	F
7777	2	1.27	52—60	1.0	Pd	0/10	73	F
3924A [b]	1	1.87	264—272	1.0	Pd	3/7	65—73	FC
7288C	5	1.52	93—102	1.2	Pd	8/2	43	M
$H35tc_2$	1		95—104	0.7	Pd	7/3	52	M
7288ctc	5	1.52	50—59	0.7	Pd	10/0	67—69	M
$H35tc_1$	1		120—129	0.7	Pd	2/8	49—50	M
3683F	1	1.87	261—270	0.6	Pd	5/5	39—40	M

Pd — Poorly differentiated; WD-Pd — Intermediate between well differentiated and poorly differentiated; WD — Well differentiated; HD — Highly differentiated; WD-HD — Intermediate between well differentiated and highly differentiated; NK — Normal karyotype.

[a] Tumor displaced by lymphoma cells.

[b] FC — Castrated female receiving testosterone.

Table 2. Transplantable hepatomas histological and biological characteristics (Cont'd)

Tumors	Inducing agent	Level mM/kg	Generations used	Months between transfers Avg.	Histological type	Metastases −/+	Chromosome number	Primary sex
(1) N-2 FdiAA								
47C	1	0.56	1—4	7.7	HD	1/3	—	M
39A	1	0.56	1—5	7.2	HD-WD	2/4	—	M
28A	1	0.56	2—5	6.0	HD	2/2	82—85	M
44	1	0.56	1—4	5.8	WD	3/1	85	M
42A	1	0.56	1—4	4.7	WD	3/1	—	M
R3B	1	0.94	3—15	4.1	WD	5/5	43	M
R7	1	0.94	4—19	2.8	WD	4/6	44	M
38B	1	0.56	2—12	2.5	WD	8/2	—	M
38A	1	0.56	1—2	2.3	WD	2/0	—	M
9108	1	0.56	20—29	2.0	WD	4/6	42	M
H35	1	0.94	55—64	1.7	WD	5/5	43—44	M
9121F	1	0.56	20—29	1.7	WD	8/2	—	M
R1	1	0.94	22—31	1.6	WD	1/9	46	M
9121	1	0.56	24—33	1.5	WD	10/0	42	M
9098	1	0.56	32—41	1.2	WD-HD	7/3	42	M
3924A[b]	1	1.87	264—272	1.0	Pd	3/7	65—73	FC
$H35tc_2$	1		95—104	0.7	Pd	7/3	52	M
$H35tc_1$	1		120—129	0.7	Pd	2/8	49—50	M
3683F	1	1.87	261—270	0.6	Pd	5/5	39—40	M
(2) N-2-FPA								
7787	2	1.27	7—14	6.3	HD-WD	8/0	44	F
7794B	2	1.27	10—17	3.1	HD	2/8	44	M
7794A	2	1.27	23—30	2.9	WD	6/1	42	M
5123C	2	1.27	71—77	2.0	WD	2/8	96	F
7793	2	1.27	21—28	1.8	WD	2/8	45	F
7795	2	1.27	29—39	1.8	WD	1/8	46—47	M
7800	2	1.27	42—48	1.7	WD	2/8	42	M
5123D	2	1.27	70—80	1.6	WD-Pd	0/10	45	F
5123A	2	1.27	80—89	1.5	WD	0/10	46	F
5123B	2	1.27	93—102	1.2	WD-Pd	4/6	46	F
5123tc	2	1.27	78—86	1.2	WD-Pd	1/9	47—49	F
7777	2	1.27	52—60	1.0	Pd	0/10	73	F
(3) 2(4'CH_3) BAF								
9618B	3	1.13	1—2	10.0	W-HD	4/0	42—44	M
9618A	3	1.13	1—5	8.0	HD	14/1	42 NK	M
9611B	3	1.13	10—16	2.5	HD-WD	2/5	42—43	M
$9618A_2$	3	1.13	4—13	1.2	Pd	6/4	41	M
(4) 2-ENAF								
8624[a]	4	1.12	12	4.7	WD-HD	—	—	M
(5) N,N'-2,7-FAA(F_6)								
7288C	5	1.52	93—102	1.2	Pd	8/2	43	M
7288ctc	5	1.52	50—59	0.7	Pd	10/0	67—69	M
(6) F-2,7-N,N'DiSuccinamine Acid								
9633	6	0.88	1—10	4.0	WD	3/2	42 NK	M
9633F	6	0.88	5—9	4.0	WD	2/2	—	M

Table 2. Transplantable hepatomas histological and biological characteristics (Cont'd)

Tumors	Inducing agent	Level mM/kg	Generations used	Months between transfers Avg.	Histological type	Metastases −/+	Chromosome number	Primary sex
(7) 2,4,6-TMA								
7316B	7	1.11	32—41	1.8	WD	4/6	55	F
7316A	7	1.11	33—42	1.6	WD	0/10	43	F
(8) 4'F-4-BAA								
8995	8	1.10	18—26	2.3	WD	0/10	43	M
8994	8	1.10	29—38	1.8	Pd	9/1	72—82	M
(9) N-F-2-Nicotinamide								
66	9	1.12	1—2	11.5	HD	2/0	42 NK	M
(10) Aflatoxin B_1								
20	10	0.005	1—3	12.6	HD-WD	3/0	—	M
21	10	0.005	1—4	10.8	HD	3/0	—	M
16	10	0.005	1—4	10.5	W-HD	3/0	42—44	M
6	10	0.005	1—5	5.5	HD-WD	5/0	44	M

[a] Tumor displaced by lymphoma cells.
[b] FC — Castrated female receiving testosterone.

carcinogen in the diet such as N-2-fluorenyldiacetamide (2-FdiAA) will usually produce a rapidly growing poorly-differentiated tumor (cf. Table 2). A low level of incorporation of this very active carcinogen for a few weeks will result in hepatomas that are well- to highly-differentiated, and slower growing. A moderately active carcinogen such as N-2-fluorenylphthalamic acid (2-FPA), however, will induce predominately well-differentiated tumors. This is illustrated in Table 2.

After many attempts by repeated experiments with the same carcinogen, we have been unable to induce identical tumors even in instances where two primary tumors have developed in the same liver. A decade ago van Potter proposed the term "minimal deviation" hepatomas to identify those slow to medium growth rate tumors that approached minimal changes from the so-called liver marker enzyme activities of normal adult rat liver [1], i. e., enzymes present predominately in the rat liver.

The first one of these transplantable hepatomas examined by Potter was one induced in our laboratory by the ingestion of a diet containing FPA designated tumor No. 5123. Since after many studies it is now clear that several of our spectrum of hepatomas do not fit Potter's concept of a "minimal deviation" hepatoma [2], therefore, it is more correct to refer to our spectrum of tumors as Morris hepatomas. We have supplied investigators throughout the world with many different lines of these transplantable hepatomas. I like to refer to the various lines as "pedigreed tumors" because we maintain very detailed records of each tumor through every transfer from its primary development up to the latest transfer.

Any given tumor line once induced seems to retain most of its histological and biological characteristics. We do not have any identical tumors, therefore, one could conclude that there may be many different primary lesions (sites) which are altered perhaps at random, because we do not induce identical tumors by the chemical carcinogens we have used. Thus, there is great diversity in these biological models, even though the hepatomas originate from liver parenchymal cells. In trying to understand the problem of cancer I believe it is necessary to examine the end product — the tumor. What better experimental system could be developed than a spectrum of tumors derived from the same cell type, e. g., the liver parenchymal cell. Normal control tissue, the adult non-tumor bearing rat liver is readily available in quantity. These full blown hepatomas, possessing different growth rates and different degrees of malignancy, are also being produced in quantity. It is, therefore, possible to compare a spectrum of these tumors with control liver to determine the presence of alterations that appear to be essential from the non-essential changes that have taken place in neoplastic liver. Fetal and regenerating liver are also easily obtained.

In neoplasia, those regulatory mechanisms that are normally present in homeostasis no longer control cell growth. Some of the alterations may result in cell death, other alterations may be insufficient to permit "uncontrolled growth" whereas changes that result in transplantable tumors have their cells sufficiently altered to support growth independent of the host. Other alterations present may be coincidential to neoplasia. It is very important to use inbred animals for inducing "minimal deviation" types of slowly growing well- to highly-differentiated transplantable tumors because the immunological competency of the highly inbred strains more closely resemble that of the primary host in which the hepatomas were induced and we believe allows cells only slightly altered to grow in the new host thus allowing propagation of somatic neoplastic cells of the "minimal deviation" type. These tumors are quite selective because they do not grow satisfactorily in other inbred strains or in non-inbred stocks of rats.

Some additional important biological and biochemical properties of our spectrum of hepatomas are summarized in Table 3. In this table the hepatomas have been conveniently separated into three groups according to their degree of differentiation as described by many morphologists [2, 4, 5, 6].

It is apparent that the rapidly growing poorly-differentiated hepatoms show a greater degree of deviation from normal than do the other two classes. Much of our

Table 3. Biological and biochemical properties of hepatomas

Hepatoma	Degree of differentiation		
Growth rate	High Very low	Well Low	Poor Rapid
Chromosome	Normal or nearly normal	Some near diploid Some near tetraploid	Abnormal
Chromosome Karyotype	Normal or nearly normal	Nearly Normal	Abnormal
Respiration	High	Moderate	Moderately low
Glycolysis	Low	Low	High
Enzyme	Few alterations	Some alterations	Many alterations
Metastases	Fewer	Variable	Variable
Deviations	Minimal	Several	Many

present understanding of neoplasia stems from those slow growing tumors which have "minimal deviation" but which can be contrasted to the more rapidly growing poorly-differentiated tumors.

One system of great importance in glucose metabolism is the glucose-ATP phosphotransferases, enzymes which transfer phosphate from ATP to glucose to form glucose-6-phosphate, and act as the portal of entry for glucose metabolism. A series of experiments by WEINHOUSE *et al.*, 1971, have produced quantitative data showing glucokinase and the three hexokinases as determined by kinetic assays [6, 7, 8].

These experiments showed that the high-glucokinase low-hexokinase pattern found in adult liver is present in the highly-differentiated hepatomas. In the poorly-differentiated hepatomas, on the other hand, there is a very high level of hexokinase and almost complete loss of glucokinase. This suggests that the glucokinase gene is suppressed with a decrease in differentiation, and the genes that code for hexokinases are activated. The poorly-differentiated, rapidly growing tumors that have high-hexokinase levels also have a high capability of glucose utilization — a high glycolytic activity.

Glucokinase is under the host hormonal, and dietary influences, and has a low affinity for glucose. This enzyme would, therefore, take up glucose only during hyperglycemia. The hexokinase isozymes, however, would use glucose at very low glucose concentration, therefore, would be functioning at maximum capacity under physiological conditions.

The high aerobic glycolysis of many tumors has been a challenging problem to cancer investigators ever since O. WARBURG, more than 50 years ago first observed that glucose utilization and lactic acid production, a process he termed glycolysis, was high anaerobically and was strikingly lowered by oxygen [9]. He termed this effect of oxygen as the Pasteur Effect. WARBURG found that the Pasteur Effect in normal tissues led to nearly complete inhibition of glycolysis, but this inhibition was only partial with tumor tissue, thus leading to a high tumor aerobic glycolysis. WARBURG regarded this respiratory impairment as a key to neoplastic transformation. This high aerobic glycolysis of many cancers has been a focal point of much experimental work on regulatory mechanisms in carbohydrate metabolism. Much attention has been directed to the activity of those enzymes which serve as sites of transphosphorylation; especially those that utilize ADP or inorganic phosphate. Respiration is coupled with the combination of ADP and Pi to yield ATP and these are the sites where glycolysis competes with respiration for these substances.

Another enzyme, pyruvate kinase plays a crucial role in the formation as well as breakdown of glucose. It is also one of the sites where ATP is formed in glycolysis and is involved in the complex regulatory mechanism known as the Pasteur Effect.

When it was found [7], that the total pyruvate kinase levels (Type I and Type II) was from 5 to 10-fold higher in the highly glycolyzing well-differentiated tumors and that the non-hepatic Type I pyruvate kinase predominately present in these rapidly growing tumors was not inhibited by high levels of ATP, and it would be expected to remain active under aerobic conditions that would inhibit the liver type enzyme.

These expectations were confirmed in model systems by intermixing glycolytic and respiratory systems from low and high glycolyzing tumors, Table 4 [10].

As shown in Table 4, broken cell preparations of poorly- and well-differentiated tumors were separated into particulate (or respiratory mitochondria) system and supernatant (glycolytic system), and the two fractions were reconstituted the glycolysis was high from the PD tumors and the preponderance of ATP was formed by glycolysis with only a small fraction by respiration. The opposite result was found for the WD tumor preparations namely, slight glycolytic ATP production and high respiratory ATP.

Table 4. Results of mixing respiratory systems from P. D. and W. D. hepatomas from WEINHOUSE *et al.* (1971)

Glycolytic system	Respiratory system	Glycolytic ATP	Respiratory ATP
P. D.	P. D.	+++++	+
W. D.	W. D.	+	+++
P. D.	W. D.	++	+++
W. D.	P. D.	+++	+

When the high glycolytic system containing high pyruvate kinase activity was mixed with the high respiratory system from a well-differentiated tumor, the respiratory system (line 3) glycolysis successfully competes for ADP and glycolytic ATP is predominate. GOSALVEZ and WEINHOUSE (personal communication) have demonstrated directly competition for ADP between purified pyruvate kinase and isolated mitochondria in the presence of phosphoenolpyruvate and a respiratory substrate. These observations suggest that the competition for ADP between pyruvate kinase and the mitochondrial apparatus for oxidative phosphorylation is an important factor in determining the magnitude of the Pasteur Effect. The high activity of isozyme I may explain the high aerobic glycolysis of tumors. These observations also document that high aerobic glycolysis is not a *sine qua non* of cancer, but rather is a phenotypic expression of a late stage in de-differentiation of cancer cells.

Synthetic and Degradative Pathways of Thymidine Utilization and the Alteration of Gene Expression in the Cancer Cell

The identification of the pattern of gene expression in cancer cells has been extensively studied by WEBER *et al.* [11], thymidine utilization and degradation in differentiating, regenerating, and neoplastic liver demonstrate that the incorporation of thymidine into DNA increases and concurrently the degradation to CO_2 decreases parallel with hepatoma growth rate. These parameters were determined simultaneously in tumor slices in an *in vitro* system. Incorporation of thymidine into DNA was very high in newborn rats. The incorporation gradually decreasing to very low levels in the adult. The incorporation of thymidine is 30-fold higher in the 1-day old rat than in the adult. While the catabolic or degradative pathway to CO_2 of thymidine occurs in the newborn rat liver, this activity increases during differentiation to an overwhelmingly higher activity than the activity of the synthetic pathway in the adult. This rise in the activity of the catabolic pathway is blocked by actinomycin. Two daily injections of actinomycin completely prevented the rise of the catabolic pathway during development. On the other hand, the administration of the drug to the slice system was ineffective on the incorporation of thymidine into DNA or the degradation of thymidine to CO_2. The increase in the catabolic pathway during development, therefore, seems to entail an increase in the biosynthesis of key enzymes, and the production of new RNA.

During the resting state in adult rat liver the ratio of the synthetic: to the degradative pathway is very low. The behavior, however, of opposing pathways of synthetic and catabolic utilization in regenerating adult liver is strikingly different [11]. Eighteen hours after partial hepatectomy, however, there was a 5-fold rise in activity of the synthetic pathway and an 18% decrease in the catabolic pathway. This imbalance reached its maximum 24 hours after operation with a 15-fold increase in the ratio, and returned to normal after 96 hours. It is possible, therefore, to unleash the genome potential in adult differentiated rat liver by partial hepatectomy. This differentiated rat liver, during regeneration, results in a rise in hepatic cell replicative function involving mitosis thereby increasing the number of cells until the preoperative state has been re-established.

The rise in enzyme synthesis following partial hepatectomy may result either from a derepression or induction of closely linked genes [11]. The "forces" that operate in a reciprocal manner in controlling the opposing pathways of thymidine utilization are capable of restoring the balance of the adult liver steady state after the regeneration reaches completion. This is shown graphically in Fig. 1.

In a series of 9 transplantable hepatomas in our spectrum that differ 15-fold in growth rate the behavior of the opposing pathways of thymidine (Tdr) utilization is illustrated in Fig. 1. It will be noted that (left side), where the percent of normal liver values are expressed, that in the very slowest growing hepatomas the incorporation of thymidine to DNA increased nearly 3-fold and in the degradative pathway of thymidine a decrease of 49% was observed. Even in the very slowest growing tumor the ratio value (right side of Fig. 1) increased 6-fold over the value observed in liver of control rats. There is an increase in the synthetic pathway of thymidine and a decrease in the activity of the catabolic pathway. The incorporation of thymidine to DNA in the fastest growing tumor in this series ($9618A_2$) increased 31-fold, whereas, the degradative pathway decreased only 0.04% of the values of normal rat liver used as controls. The ratio, however, $\frac{\text{Tdr to} \rightarrow \text{DNA}}{\text{Tdr to} \rightarrow CO_2}$ increased 140,000-fold.

The data presented in these charts emphasize the importance of ratios of activities of opposing enzyme and pathways as indicator of links between replicative, translative, and transcriptive expression of the altered genome in neoplasia.

Further support for altered gene expression in neoplasia has been reported by Elford *et al.* [12], who found a high correlation in nucleic acid metabolism between ribonucleotide reductase activity and growth rate, a similar positive correlation was recognized by Ove *et al.* [13], for DNA polymerase activity.

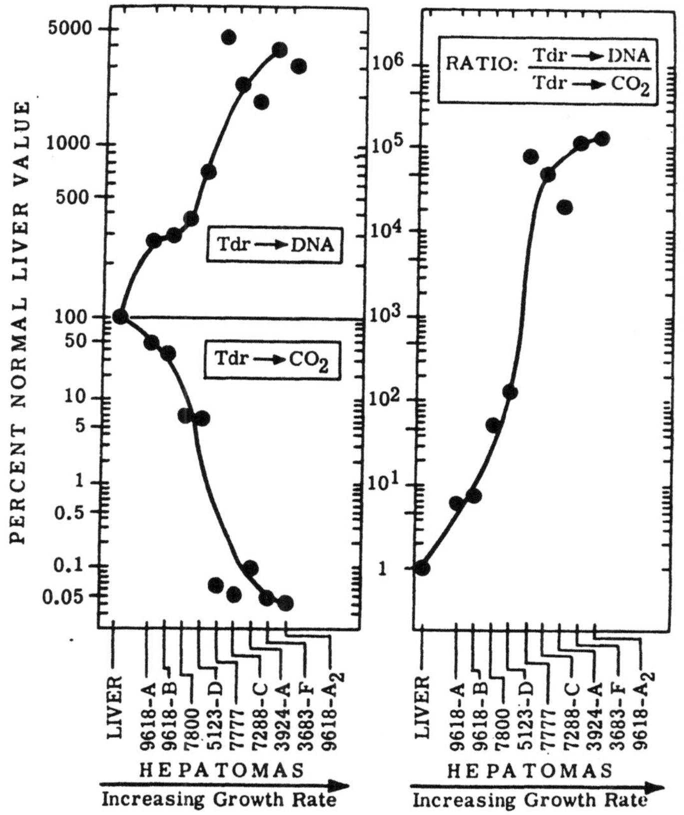

Fig. 1

The regenerating liver grows at a rate comparable to that of the faster growing hepatomas, however, the imbalance that is linked to proliferation rate is much more pronounced in the hepatomas than in the regenerating liver. These alterations noted in the hepatomas, therefore, appear to be specific to the tumor system. In the very young rat there is a high synthetic utilization of thymidine but a strong degradative pathway is also operating simultaneously. Thus, the striking imbalance that is found in thymidine metabolism in the hepatomas that is correlated with tumor growth rate seems to be specific to the neoplastic alteration in gene expression and supports the Molecular Correlation Concept of WEBER and LEA [14].

Loss of Feedback Control in Hepatomas

The only parameter examined so far that is uniformly altered in all neoplastic liver is the loss of feedback control noted by SIPERSTEIN *et al.* in all species so far examined. As you know, dietary or exogenous cholesterol in mammals and fish markedly suppresses cholesterol synthesis in the liver.

SIPERSTEIN and FAGAN [15], showed that the feedback control of cholesterol synthesis is specifically at the enzymatic step responsible for the conversion of

3-hydroxy-3-methyl-glutarate to mevalonate. A number of investigators [16], have found that the conversion of labelled 3-hydroxy-3-methyl-glutaryl-coenzyme A (HMG-CoA) to mevalonate is inhibited by exogenous cholesterol. These observations uphold the view that the primary site of cholesterol feedback control is at the reaction responsible for the synthesis of mevalonate.

SIPERSTEIN *et al.* [17], have reported that in striking contrast to the presence of the cholesterol feedback reaction noted above in normal liver cells, the feedback control is lost when the hepatocyte becomes malignant. SIPERSTEIN *et al.* [18] have demonstrated this deletion in all hepatomas regardless of species, degree of differentiation, or method of induction of the hepatoma. Furthermore, this observation is the only known example of a consistent deletion of a feedback system in tumors and it may indicate that the disturbance of the enzyme site responsible for the synthesis of mevalonate could represent a characteristic of neoplasia. This concept is supported by the recent report of SIPERSTEIN *et al.*, that this feedback lesion of cancer is localized at the enzyme mevalonate: NADP oxidreductase (acylating CoA) hydroxymethylglutaryl CoA reductase. The data for two hepatomas are illustrated in the following Table 5 [22].

Table 5. Feedback control of HMG-CoA reductase in normal liver and 2 hepatomas

Experiment	Tissue	Treatment	Cholesterol synthesis	HMG-CoA reductase [a]
A	Liver	—	90	0.77 ± 0.26
	Liver	5% Cholesterol	1.6	0.007± 0.01
	Hepatoma 9121	—	91	1.34 ± 0.32
	Hepatoma 9121	5% Cholesterol	192	1.69 ± 0.38
B	Liver	—	—	2.21 ± 0.29
	Liver	5% Cholesterol	—	0.18 ± 0.05
	Hepatoma 9121	—	—	2.00 ± 0.25
	Hepatoma 9121	5% Cholesterol	—	1.59 ± 0.26
C	Liver	—	—	1.14 ± 0.10
	Liver	5% Cholesterol	—	0.11 ± 0.01
	Hepatoma 3924A	—	—	4.7 ± 0.34
	Hepatoma 3924A	5% Cholesterol	—	4.5 ± 0.25

[a] Conversion by microsomes isolated from 800 mg. of liver, cf. SIPERSTEIN *et al.*, 1971.

While these data localize the biochemical site of this feedback defect in neoplasia they give no direct information as to whether this lesion represents an alteration in HMG-CoA reductase, the formation of isozymes, a derangement in either transcriptional or translational control of the synthesis of this enzyme, or the formation or alteration an inhibitor of the reaction.

Diversity Among Hepatomas

Our spectrum of hepatomas except for loss of feedback control in cholesterol synthesis, exhibit a profound diversity of metabolic patterns. Some of the key enzymes in carbohydrate and nucleic acid metabolism appear to be correlated with growth rate and the degree of differentiation. The not very precise measure of growth rate we use seems to be highly correlated with more precise biochemical parameters, to name two; thymidine incorporation [11], and ribonucleotide reductase [12]. There are many other parameters not correlated with growth.

Of special interest are the responses of a spectrum of 9 hepatomas, 7 of which were diploid tumors, to the activity of four enzymes plus glycogen [19, 20]. These enzymes were compared at three dietary protein levels and controlled feeding conditions of either 8 + 16 or 8 + 40 hours, i.e., eight hours with food and 16 or 40 hours without food. The two most "minimal" hepatomas in this spectrum are 9618A and 9633. These tumors according to NOWELL *et al.* [21], have a normal karyotype. Only 9618A is completely lacking tyrosine transminase but it is the only hepatoma with nearly a normal amount of glycogen. Glycogen is absent or very low in all the other hepatomas. Serine dehydratase is missing in several hepatomas. The enzyme activities of the host livers are affected to a much less extent.

The adult liver may not be the best tissue for comparison but as pointed out earlier neither is regenerating or neonatal liver wholely satisfactory. Are the primary hepatomas induced in a single immature hepatocyte whose further maturation is blocked as suggested by POTTER? The resulting hepatoma if it grows in the new host may not be able to carry out the maturation sequence and might become a permanently altered clone that is recognized as liver neoplasia [20].

Summary

A review is given about the histological and biochemical characteristics of the so-called minimal deviation hepatomas. Some key enzymes in carbohydrate and nucleic acid metabolism appear to be correlated with growth rate and the degree of differentiation. The most "minimal" hepatomas have a normal karyotype. In the other hepatomas with aneuploid chromosome numbers, glycogen and four enzymes of the carbohydrate metabolism are absent or very low.

References

1. POTTER, V. R.: Cancer Res. **21**, 1331 (1961).
2. MORRIS, H. P., WAGNER, B. P.: Meth. Cancer Res. **4**, 125 (1968); Ed.: H. BUSCH. New York: Academic Press, Inc.
3. REUBER, M. D.: Ganan Mongr. 1, 43 (1966).
4. MIYAJI, H., MORRIS, H. P., WAGNER, B. P.: Meth. Cancer Res. **4**, 153 (1968); Ed.: H. BUSCH. New York: Academic Press, Inc.
5. HRUBAN, Z., MORRIS, H. P., MOCHIZUKI, Y., MERANZE, D. R., SESSORS, A.: Cancer Res. **31**, 752 (1971).
6. WEINHOUSE, S., SHATTON, J. B., CRISS, W. E., FARINA, F. A., MORRIS, H. P.: Gann Mongr. **13**, 36 (1972).
7. WEINHOUSE, S., SHATTON, J. B., CRISS, W. E., MORRIS, H. P.: Molecular Forms of Enzymes. Paris: Conference on Molecular Pathology 1971.
8. FARINA, F. A., ADELMAN, R. C., MORRIS, H. P., LO, C. H., WEINHOUSE, S.: Cancer Res. **28**, 1897 (1968).
9. WARBURG O.: London: Arnold Constable 1930.
10. SHATTON J. B., MORRIS, H. P., WEINHOUSE, S.: Cancer Res. **29**, 1161 (1969).
11. FERDINANDUS J. A., MORRIS, H. P., WEBER, G.: Cancer Res. **31**, 550 (1971).
12. ELFORD, H. L., FREESE, M., PASSAMANI, E., MORRIS, H. P.: J. biol. Chem. **245**, 5228 (1970).

13. OVE, P., LASZLO, J., JENKINS, M. D., MORRIS, H. P.: Cancer Res. **29**, 1557 (1969).
14. WEBER, G., LEA, M. A.: Meth. Cancer Res. **2**, 523 (1967); Ed.: H. BUSCH.
15. SIPERSTEIN, M. D., FAGAN, V. M.: J. biol. Chem. **241**, 206 (1960).
16. SIPERSTEIN, M. D.: Current Topics in Cellular Regulation. Eds. E. STADTMAN and B. HORECKER. New York: Academic Press 1970, Vol. 2, p. 65.
17. SIPERSTEIN, M. D., FAGAN, V. M., MORRIS, H. P.: Cancer Res. **26**, 7 (1966).
18. SIPERSTEIN, M. D., GYDE, A. M., MORRIS, H. P.: Proc. nat. Acad. Sci. (Wash.) **68**, 315 (1971).
19. POTTER, V. R., WATANABE, M., PITOT, H. C., MORRIS, H. P.: Cancer Res. **29**, 55 (1969).
20. POTTER, V. R., WATANABE, M.: Int'l. Leukemia — Lymphoma Conf. Proc. Philadelphia, Pa.: Lea and Febiger Pub. Co. 1968, p. 33.
21. NOWELL, P. C., MORRIS, H. P., POTTER, V. R.: Cancer Res. **27**, 1565 (1967).
22. BRICKER, L. A., MORRIS, H. P., SIPERSTEIN, M. D.: J. clin. Invest. **51**, 206 (1972).

Carcinogen-induced Cellular Thesaurismoses and Neoplastic Cell Transformation

P. BANNASCH

It has been known for a long time from human pathology that many tumors contain cells which store polysaccharides or lipids. So far such pathological storage phenomena have been interpreted as a consequence of the neoplastic cell transformation and to be related to the general disturbance of tumor cell metabolism. Experimental investigations of the genesis of epithelial liver and kidney tumors have shown, however, that cellular thesaurismoses are mainly characteristic of the preneoplastic phase (BANNASCH *et al.* 1964—1972). In the development of certain tumors they seem to be an inevitable step, indicating a basic alteration of cell metabolism. During cellular transformation there is usually a gradual reduction in the amount of the stored substances. Therefore, thesaurismoses in tumors can be considered as relicts of the preneoplastic phase. Four examples will be used to illustrate this concept.

1. Hepatocellular Glycogenosis and Hepatoma Development

Histochemical and electron microscopical investigations of hepatocarcinogenesis in nitrosomorpholine(NNM)-intoxicated rats have shown that the appearance of hepatomas is regularly preceded by hepatocellular glycogenosis persisting for weeks or even months (BANNASCH and MÜLLER 1964; BANNASCH 1967, 1968). An unusual accumulation of glycogen in the cytoplasm of hepatocytes has also been observed following treatment with numerous other hepatotropic carcinogens, such as diethylnitrosamine (SCHAUER and KUNZE 1968; FRIEDRICH-FREKSA *et al.* 1969), dimethylaminoazobenzene (FORGET and DAOUST 1970), 2-fluorenylacetamide (EPSTEIN *et al.* 1967) and aflatoxin (NEWBERNE and WOGAN 1968). This indicates an obligatory development of hepatocellular glycogenosis after carcinogenic liver poisons.

The increased glycogen content is the main reason for the long-known enlargement and clearing of the carcinogen-intoxicated hepatocytes (Fig. 1). Electronmicroscopically the glycogen particles are found mainly in the cytoplasmic matrix. In some storage cells large glycogen portions are enclosed in autophagic vacuoles and become finely granular, probably as a consequence of lysosomal degradation. Other components of the cytoplasm, especially the basophilic bodies, are often pushed towards the periphery of the cell or into the vicinity of the nucleus, and the amount of basophilic bodies (ergastoplasm) per unit volume of cytoplasm is then markedly reduced. The fine structure of the ergastoplasm, however, invariably remains almost unchanged.

In addition to the dislocation and relative reduction of the granular endoplasmic reticulum (ergastoplasm) a proliferation of the agranular reticulum (AR) takes place in many storage cells. The proliferated smooth membranes are usually closely associated with glycogen particles. The cause and the significance of the membrane proliferation is largely obscure. Following the ideas of Porter and Bruni (1959) we assume that it is linked directly or indirectly to the alterations of intracellular glycogen metabolism. An enhancement of glycogen and agranular membranes also exists in many hepatocytes ("X-cells") which at first sight appear normal, but which actually show a 1,5—2 fold enlargement of their cells areas (Bannasch *et al.* 1972).

After continuous application of a 12 mg% NNM-solution (drinking water) the excess glycogen storage develops within a few weeks (Bannasch and Müller 1964): "Clear" storage cells can be observed after a fortnight in the peripheral and intermediate regions of the liver lobules. Within 12—16 weeks multiple glycogen storage foci develop in all experimental animals. These foci probably correspond to the "areas of hyperplasia" which, according to Reuber (1966), are not yet transplantable.

The transformation of "areas of hyperplasia" into the so called "hyperplastic nodules", which are nowadays generally accepted to be direct precursors of hepatomas, has been well documented (see Farber 1963; Reuber 1966; Bannasch 1968). At the cellular level the transformation into hepatomas is characterized by a gradual reduction of the glycogen which was initially stored in excess and with a concomitant increase in the number of ribosomes (Bannasch 1967, 1968). This manifests itself light microscopically in an increase in cytoplasmic basophilia long known as "chromatogenesis" (Fig. 1). The hypertrophied AR is largely transformed during this process into an atypically granular reticulum by the addition of ribosomes. Furthermore there is often a transitory accumulation of fine or coarse fat droplets. The endpoint of cellular transformation is marked by a deficiency of glycogen, fat and AR, together with a relatively high content of ribosomes or ergastoplasm. In livers of diethylnitrosamine-intoxicated rats such cells show an increase in both cytoplasmic RNA content (Hobik and Grundmann 1962) and RNA synthesis (Oehlert and Hartje 1963).

The best information on the relation of carcinogen-induced glycogen storage cells to hepatoma cells is gained from "stop" experiments, in which the carcinogenic treatment is discontinued after several weeks. While nonspecific toxic parenchymal lesions are reversible after the cessation of poisoning, hepatocellular glycogenosis persists for several weeks or months, gradually disappearing only during the formation of the actual hepatomas (Bannasch 1968; Bannasch *et al.* 1972). Thus the glycogen reduction and ribosomal enrichment, characteristic of cellular transformation, are not an immediate consequence of the intoxication, but reactions of the cell to the primary carcinogenic lesion.

The nature of this initial cell alteration remains unclear. Toxic deficiencies of glycogenolytic enzymes, such as glucose-6-phosphatase or phosphorylase, have been discussed as possible causes of the preneoplastic hepatocellular glycogenosis (Bannasch and Müller 1964; Epstein *et al.* 1967; Bannasch 1968; Schauer and Kunze 1968; Friedrich-Freksa *et al.* 1969). However, this has not been conclusively proved. The biochemical mechanism responsible for the loss of glycogen is also unknown. We have suggested that it may be related to the beginning of Warburg-type glycolysis

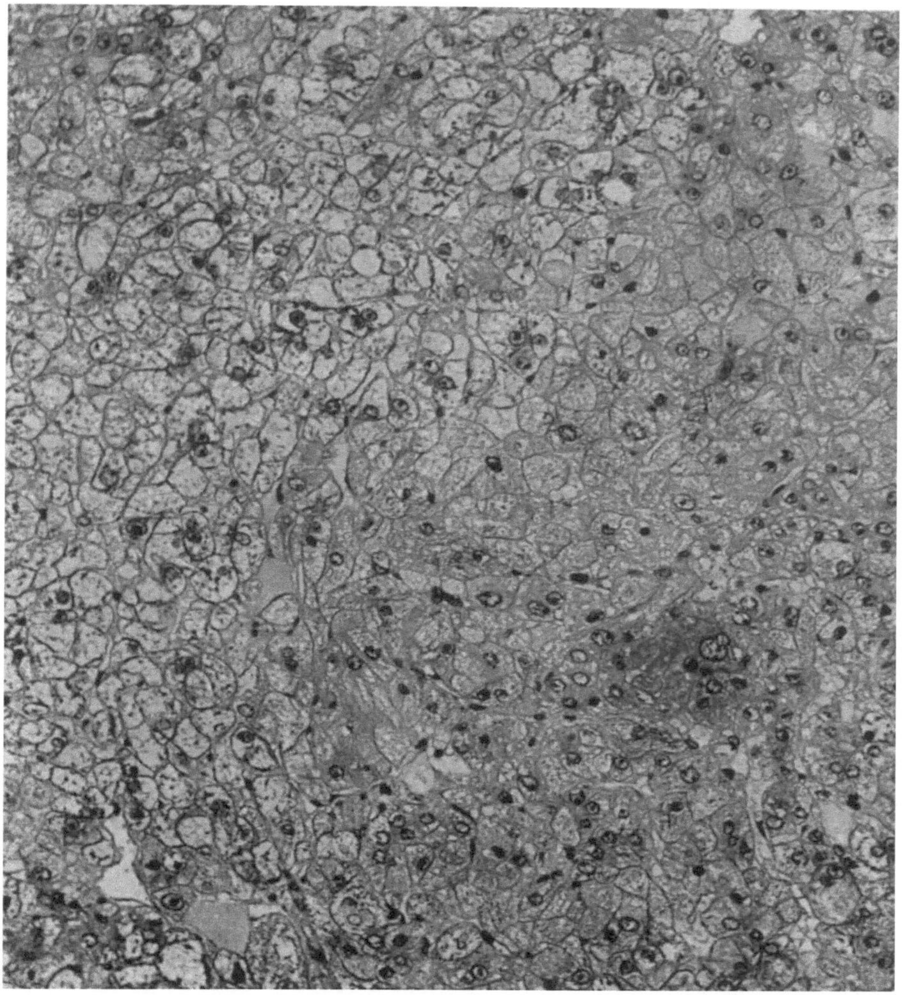

Fig. 1. Transition of a NNM-induced hepatocellular glycogenosis (left) into a glycogen-poor hepatoma (right). Rat liver. HE. 200 : 1

(BANNASCH 1968), which seems to be in accordance with the recent results of HRUBAN *et al.* (1971). They found that quickly growing hepatomas with intense glycolytic activity are almost always free of glycogen, while slowly growing tumors with low glycolytic activity are often relatively rich in glycogen (see also WEBER 1968).

2. Tubular Glycogenosis and the Genesis of Clear Cell ("Hypernephroid") Kidney Tumors

A second type of epithelial tumor, the genesis of which is accompanied by pathological glycogen storage, is the clear cell kidney tumor (Fig. 2 a—c). In NNM-

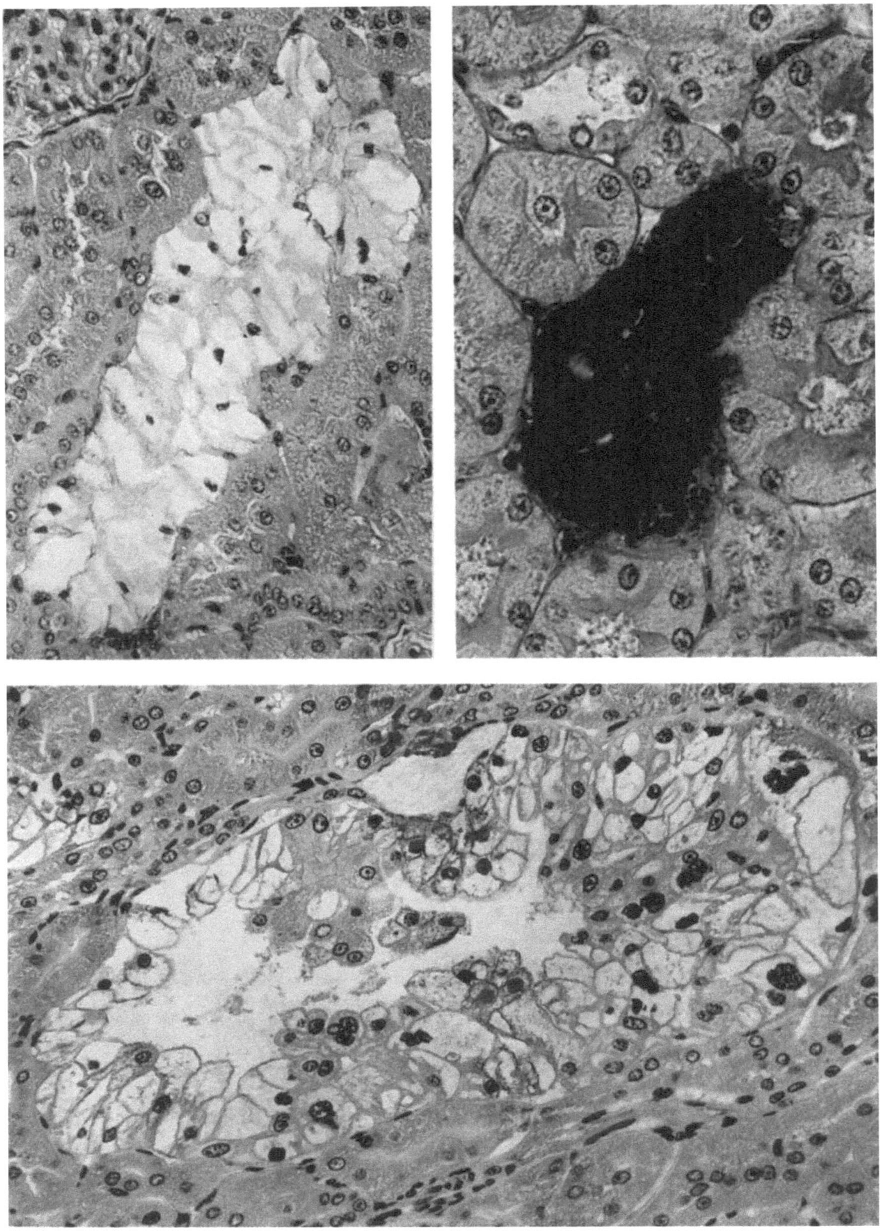

Fig. 2 a—c. NNM-induced tubular glycogenosis and tumor development in rat kidney: a glycogen storage tubule after staining with HE: characteristically clear cells with condensed nuclei. 360 : 1, b Storage tubule after demonstration of the glycogen by the PAS-reaction. Tri-PAS. 550 : 1, c Beginning of the neoplastic transformation of a glycogen storage tubule: transformation of many storage cells into glycogen-poor tumor cells, prominent atypicalities of cells and nuclei. HE. 350 : 1 (from Bannasch, P., and Schacht, U.: Verh. Dtsch. Ges. Path. **54**, 464, 1970)

intoxicated rats the tumor originates from tubules with excessive glycogen storage (BANNASCH and SCHACHT 1968; 1970). Similar results were obtained by ITO *et al.* (1966) and by HARD and BUTLER (1971) in rats poisoned with dimethylnitrosamine. After NNM treatment the PAS-positive glycogen storage tubules develop mainly in "stop" experiments, some weeks after the discontinuation of the carcinogen (Fig. 2 b). After staining with hematoxilin-eosin typical clear cells with condensed nuclei are seen (Fig. 2 a). Occasional remnants of the brush border indicate that the storage tubules are derived from the proximal nephron. The transformation into tumors can be followed through all its stages (BANNASCH and SCHACHT 1970). It is accompanied by the transformation of many glycogen storage cells into glycogen-poor or glycogen-free tumor cells (Fig. 2 c).

Electronmicroscopically the storage cells show a considerable amount of monoparticular glycogen, but only a few mitochondria and ergastoplasmic profiles (Fig. 3). In addition to the typical clear cells the tumors also contain ribosome-rich basophilic and mitochondria-rich acidophilic cells. Of particular interest is the occurence of lipoid-storing cells in the "hypernephroid" tumors (Fig. 4). The lipoids form membrane-enclosed osmiophilic bodies often showing a concentrically layered, or a parallely arranged, pattern of dark and light lines with a periodicity of 50—70 Å. Similar structures are found in the central nervous system in association with certain human storage diseases, such as gargyolism. In this case they contain predominantly gangliosides (glycolipids) but also cholesterol and phospholipids (see ALEU *et al.* 1965).

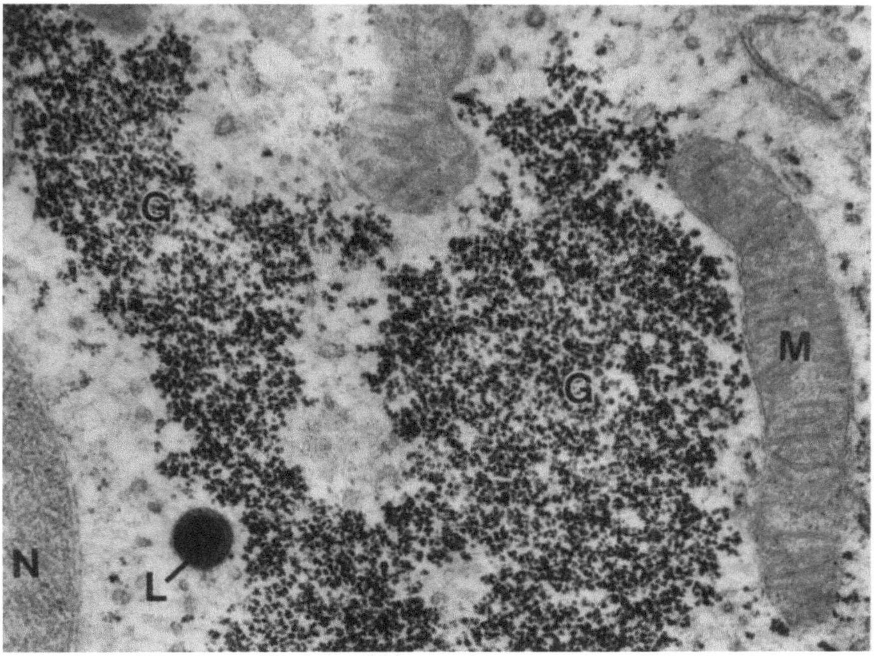

Fig. 3. Portion of a glycogen storage cell of a NNM-induced renal tumor (rat): large aggregate of monoparticular glycogen (G), nucleus (N), mitochondria (M). Lead hydroxide 25 000 : 1 (from BANNASCH, P., and SCHACHT, U.: Verh. Dtsch. Ges. Path. **54**, 464, 1970)

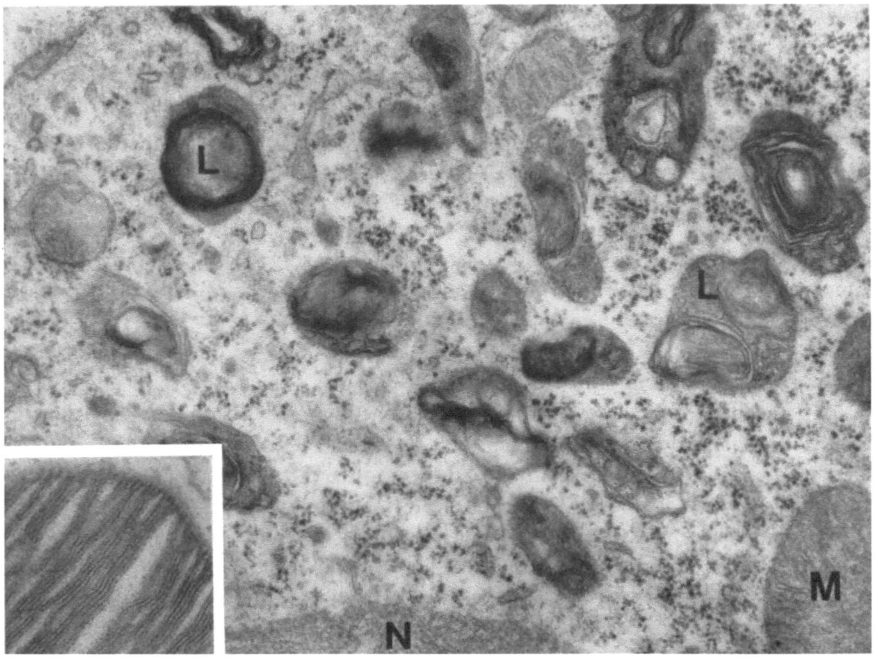

Fig. 4. Portion of a lipoid storage cell of a NNM-induced renal tumor (rat): many lipoid bodies (L), mitochondria (M), nucleus (N). Lead hydroxide 23 000 : 1. — Inset: Portion of a lipoid body showing a regular pattern of dark and light lines (period: 50—70 Å). Lead hydroxide. 80 000 : 1 (from BANNASCH, P., and SCHACHT, U.: Verh. Dtsch. Ges. Path. **54**, 464, 1970)

Our interpretation of the tubular glycogen storage cell being a precancerous cell is in good agreement with conclusions drawn by APITZ (1944) from his extensive investigations of human renal tumors. Years ago APITZ already supported the idea that the clear cells were not the carriers of malignancy but precursors of glycogen-poor or glycogen-free renal cancer cells.

3. Tubular Mucopolysaccharidosis and the Genesis of Basophilic Kidney Tumors

Treatment with NNM, under the same experimental conditions which lead to clear cell kidney tumors, often also results in the development of intensly basophilic renal adenomas (BANNASCH *et al.* 1971). We consider "chromophobe" tubules, which probably belong to the proximal nephron to be the tissue of origin of these tumors (Fig. 5a). The chromophobe tubules store excessive amounts of substances which give a positive Hale-reaction (Fig. 5b) and stain with Alcian blue, and which are therefore concluded to be acid mucopolysaccharides. As revealed by electron microscopy the cells of such tubules possess many cytoplasmic vacuoles which appear in large areas to be almost empty (Fig. 6). These regions are probably the main storage sites of acid mucopolysaccharides (see ROMEN and BANNASCH 1972). This assumption is supported by the fact that various authors have found similar vacuoles

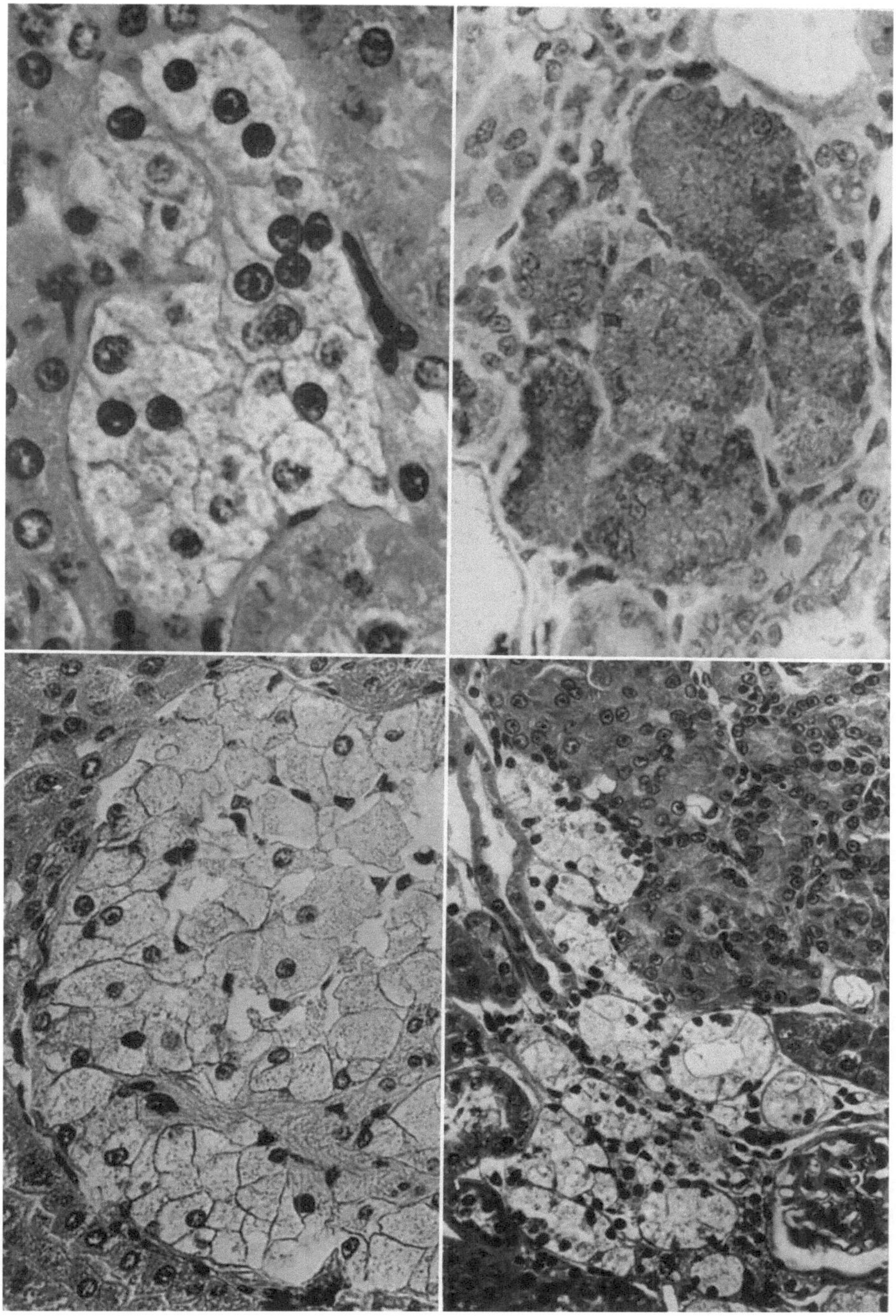

Fig. 5 a—d. NNM-induced tubular mucopolysaccharidosis and tumor development in rat kidney: a mucopolysaccharide storage tubule after staining with HE showing characteristic "chromophobe" cells with a light cytoplasm. 780 : 1, b storage tubule after demonstration of the mucopolysaccharides by the Hale-reaction. 425 : 1, c Portion of a "chromophobe" microadenoma. HE. 425 : 1, d "chromophobe" tubule in the immediate vicinity of a tubular basophilic adenoma. HE 3000 : 1 (from BANNASCH, P. *et al.*: Verh. Dtsch. Ges. Path. **55,** 665, 1971)

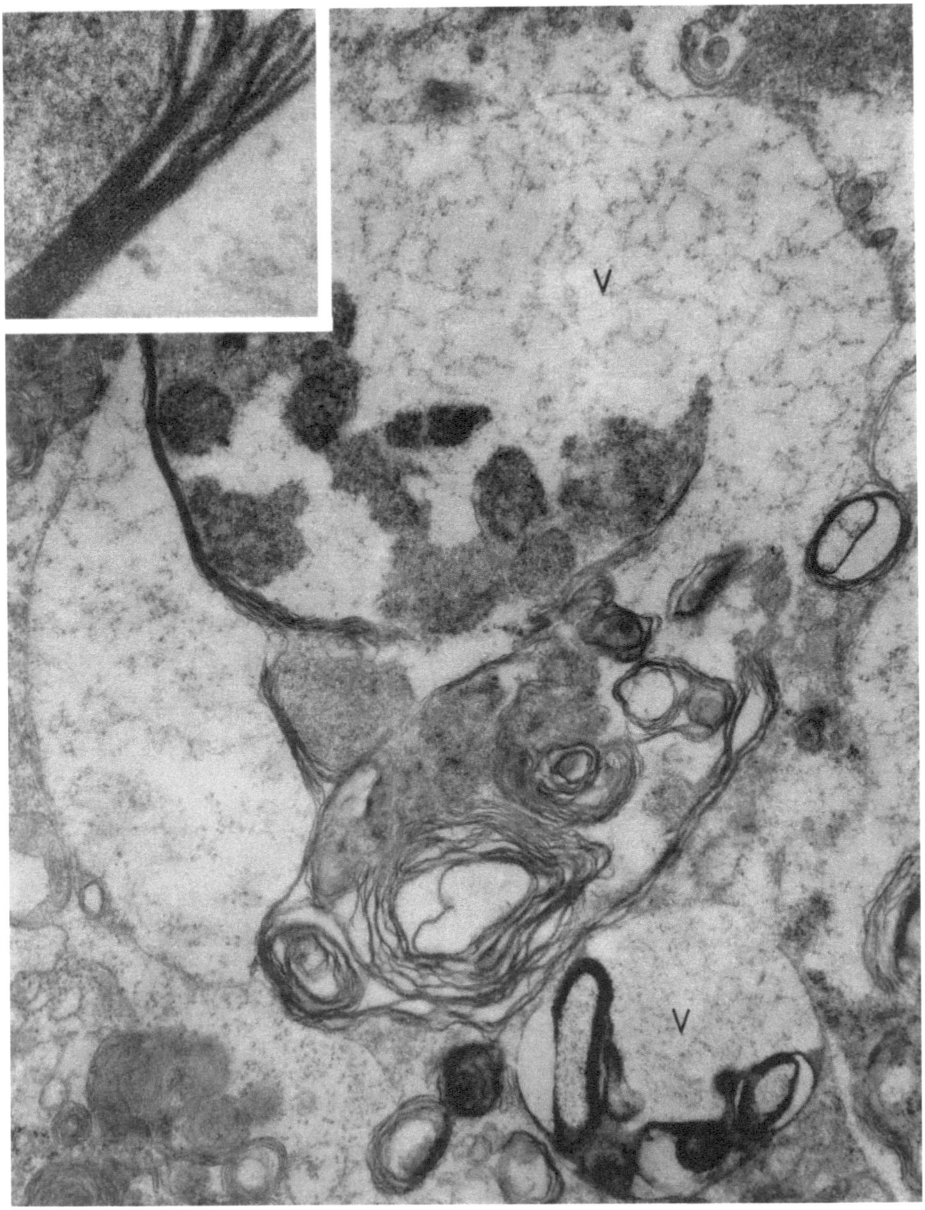

Fig. 6. Storage vacuoles (V) in tubule epithelia of the NNM-intoxicated rat kidney: large nearly empty areas and partly lamellar arranged osmiophilic material. Lead hydroxide. 24 000 : 1. — Inset: lipoid component of the storage vacuoles showing a regular pattern of dark and light lines. Lead hydroxide. 110 000 : 1

associated with certain human mucopolysaccharidoses in several organs, including the kidney. Many vacuoles of the chromophobe tubules are partly filled with lipoids which exhibit the same characteristic stripey pattern as the previously mentioned lipoids of clear cell tumors. Mixed vacuoles of this type are also known from human storage diseases and are grouped together with lysosomes (see RESIBOIS *et al.* 1970).

The relationship of the mucopolysaccharide-storing tubules to tumor genesis is supported by various morphological results. Most convincing is the occurrence of chromophobe mucopolysaccharide-loaded microtumors (Fig. 5c). Such tumors are very rare, however, since most storage cells are obviously transformed into basophilic cells as tumor development starts. We draw this conclusion from the frequent appearance of slightly basophilic, but still strongly Hale-positive tubules, on the one hand, and the close topographical interrelation of many chromophobe tubules to basophilic tumors (Fig. 5 d), on the other hand. In the latter case all intermediate stages between strongly Hale-positive tubules and weakly reacting tumor areas can be observed.

It seems justified, therefore, to assume that a "tubular mucopolysaccharidosis" occurs as a prestage of most basophilic kidney tumors. The final basophilic tumor cells are characterized in their fine structure mainly by a relative abundance of free and membrane-bound ribosomes as well as by many Golgi complexes. A rudimentary brush border sometimes indicates, even at this late stage, their origin from proximal tubular epithelia (see HARD and BUTLER 1970).

4. Cholangiolar Mucopolysaccharidosis and Cholangioma Development

Another tumor type, the genesis of which is linked to cytochemically demonstrable alterations in mucopolysaccharide metabolism is cystic cholangioma (BANNASCH and REISS 1970; 1971). In the liver of the NNM-intoxicated rat this tumor type appears particularly in "stop" experiments after a short application of high doses of carcinogen. Three distinct stages can be identified during its development. In the first stage, as an immediate consequence of toxic liver parenchymal necrosis which often reachs the periportal areas, there is a vigorous proliferation of bile duct epithelia (oval cells) and mesenchymal cells with subsequent fibrosis. In most animals this leads to a rearrangement of the liver parenchyma and to the development of multiple foci of cholangiofibrosis within a few weeks. In the second stage, as is shown particularly in "stop" experiments no further growth of the cholangiofibrosis occurs. There is, however, a conversion of the initially oval or cubic bile duct epithelia into cylindrical cells, which produce and secrete abundant mucus substances. These give positive PAS or Hale-reactions and stain with Alcian blue, which indicates that they contain neutral as well as acid mucopolysaccharides. Therefore, we call this pathologic alteration "cholangiolar mucopolysaccharidosis".

Electronmicroscopically the mucopolysaccharides are found within cytoplasmic vacuoles (BANNASCH and BERGEEST, unpublished observations). The increase in mucus production by the bile ducts, which has been described for several other hepatotropic carcinogens (see BANNASCH and REISS 1971), starts in some animals within a fortnight of the NNM-intoxication. It progresses during the experiment even without further poisoning, until, after some months, it occupies nearly all the cholangiofibrotic areas. In the third stage, which is reached after a latent period of several

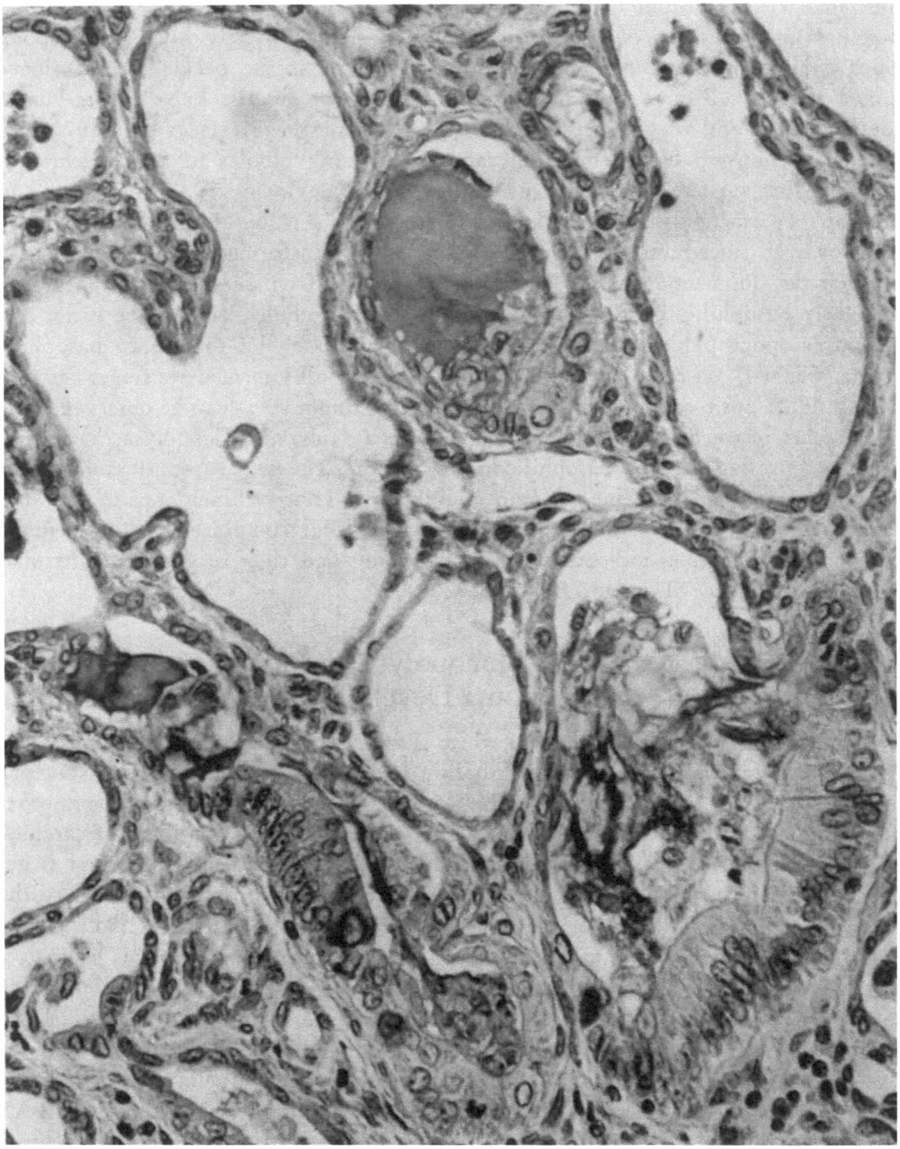

Fig. 7. Transition of mucous cholangiofibrosis in mucus free cholangioma cysts in NNM-intoxicated rats: partly cylindrical, partly flat epithelium in the mucus containing ducts. Only flat epithelia in the mucus free cysts. Tri-PAS. 450 : 1

weeks or months, the mucous cholangiofibrosis gives rise to multicystic cholangioma (Fig. 7). The cylindric mucus producing epithelia now become regularly flattened and no longer secrete mucus substances. Sometimes the typical pattern of a polycystic liver disease is observed. The electron microscope shows a richness in free and membrane bound ribosomes in the flat cells of the cysts.

Summary and Conclusions

From the comparative observation of the genesis of 4 different types of experimental liver and kidney tumors three points should be emphasized:

1. The appearance of all 4 types of epithelial tumor is preceded by a carcinogen-induced thesaurismosis. The main storage substances are polysaccharides (glycogen and mucopolysaccharides) followed by neutral fat and lipoids (glycolipids?). As revealed by histochemical and morphological methods, the focal pathological storage of these substances is, at the cellular level, very similar to the generalized alterations well known from certain human storage diseases. One should mention in this context that, in human pathology 6 cases of inborn hepatorenal glycogenosis have been described which were complicated by the appearance of hepatocellular tumors 7—19 years after birth (see BANNASCH and KLINGE 1971, SPYCHER and GITZELMANN 1971). There are also a very few examples of the combination of human mucopolysaccharidosis and tumors (SUSCHKE and KUNZE 1971).

2. As a rule the different carcinogen-induced thesaurismoses gradually disappear again during neoplastic cell transformation. At the present time it is not clear whether they are merely an accompaniment of, or a necessary prerequisite for, cellular transformation. However, the frequency of these storage phenomena in the preneoplastic cells closely examined so far indicates a more generalized pathogenetic principle. Since the stored substances are mostly polysaccharides it seems reasonable to assume an association with the development of Warburg-type glycolysis.

3. Cytologically different tumor types obviously also have a different cytogenesis. On the one hand, this statement leads us to a more profound understandment of the morphological and biological variety of tumors and, on the other hand, it opens new aspects for the diagnoses and differentiation of preneoplastic lesions.

References

ALEU, F. P., TERRY, R. D., ZELLWEGER, H.: J. Neuropath. exp. Neurol. **24**, 304 (1965).
APITZ, K.: Virchows Arch. path. Anat. **311**, 360 (1944).
BANNASCH, P.: Verh. dtsch. Ges. Path. **51**, 343 (1967).
BANNASCH, P.: Recent Results in Cancer Research, Vol. 19. Berlin-Heidelberg-New York: Springer 1968.
BANNASCH, P., KLINGE, O.: Virchows Arch. Abt. A path. Anat. **352**, 157 (1971).
BANNASCH, P., MÜLLER, H.-A.: Arzneimittel-Forsch. **14**, 805 (1964).
BANNASCH, P., PAPENBURG, J., ROSS, W.: Z. Krebsforsch. **77**, 108 (1972).
BANNASCH, P., REISS, W.: Naturwissenschaften **57**, 46 (1970).
BANNASCH, P., REISS, W.: Z. Krebsforsch. **76**, 193 (1971).
BANNASCH, P., SCHACHT, U.: Virchows Arch. Abt. B Zellpath. **1**, 95 (1968).
BANNASCH, P., SCHACHT, U.: Verh. dtsch. Ges. Path. **54**, 464 (1970).
BANNASCH, P., SCHACHT, U., WEIDNER, R., STORCH, E.: Verh. dtsch. path. Ges. **55**, 665 (1971).
EPSTEIN, SH., ITO, N., MERKOW, L., FARBER, E.: Cancer Res. **27**, 1702 (1967).
FARBER, E.: Advanc. Cancer Res. **7**, 383 (1963).
FORGET, A., DAOUST, R.: Int. J. Cancer **5**, 404 (1970).
FRIEDRICH-FREKSA, H., GÖSSNER W., BÖRNER, P.: Z. Krebsforsch. **72**, 226 (1969).
HARD, G. C., BUTLER, W. H.: Cancer Res. **30**, 2796 (1970).
HARD, G. C., BUTLER, W. H.: Cancer Res. **31**, 1496 (1971).
HOBIK, H. P., GRUNDMANN, E.: Beitr. path. Anat. **127**, 25 (1962).
HRUBAN, Z., MORRIS, H. P., MOCHIZUKI, Y., MERANZE, D. R., SLESERS, A.: Cancer Res. **31**, 752 (1971).

ITO, N., JOHUO, I., MARUGAMI, M., KONISHI, Y., HIASA, Y.: Gann **57**, 595 (1966).
NEWBERNE, P. M., WOGAN, G. N.: Cancer Res. **28**, 770 (1968).
OEHLERT, W., HARTJE, J.: Beitr. path. Anat. **128**, 376 (1963).
PORTER, K. R., BRUNI, C.: Cancer Res. **19**, 997 (1959).
RESIBOIS, A., TONDEUR, M., MOCKEL, S., DUSTIN, P.: Int. Rev. exp. Path. **9**, 93 (1970).
REUBER, M. D.: Gann Monograph **1**, 43 (1966).
ROMEN, W., BANNASCH, P.: Virchows Arch. Abt. B. Zellpath. **10**, 51 (1972).
SCHAUER, A., KUNZE, E.: Z. Krebsforsch. **70**, 252 (1968).
SPYCHER, M. A., GITZELMANN, R.: Virchows Arch. Abt. B Zellpath. **8**, 133 (1971).
SUSCHKE, J., KUNZE, D.: Dtsch. med. Wschr. **96**, 1941 (1971).
WEBER, G.: Naturwissenschaften **55**, 418 (1968).

Experimental Intestinal Carcinogenesis and Polyp Development in Rats and Mice

B. WIEBECKE

1,2-dimethylhydrazine (DMH), the carcinogen used in this experiment is characterized by marked organotropy and certainty of tumor production in the small and large intestine of rats (DRUCKREY *et al.*, 1967). It is also active in mice (WIEBECKE *et al.*, 1969).

The present experiment was carried out with 150 adult female Wistar rats and 40 adult NMRI mice. DMH was injected subcutaneously in aqueous solution. One group of rats received 14 mg, and the other group 21 mg DMH/kg body weight/week. The mice were treated with only 14 mg DMH/kg body weight/week as the LD50 in mice is considerably lower than in rats. Animals were killed periodically from the 3rd month of the experiment onwards, in order to obtain as many precursory lesions as possible. Forty minutes before they were killed the animals received an intraperitoneal injection of tritiated thymidine at a dose of 2 μC/gram body weight.

After an induction period of 200 days and a total dose of about 300 mg DMH/kg tumors of the bowels were found in every case. On the average the tumor induction time was longer in those animals which had received the lower single dose.

Species-specific as well as dosage-dependent differences were observed in the localisation of tumors. Rats often showed isolated short-stalked polyps within the large intestine, whereas mice more often tended to develop broad based and widespread tumors. In the large intestine of rats tumors were distributed uniformly, whereas in mice a preponderance in the descending colon and rectum was observed.

In rats treated with 14 mg DMH/kg tumors of the small intestine were rare compared with those of the colon. In the group treated with 21 mg DMH/kg their number rose considerably. Small bowel tumors mainly affected the duodenum, and only a few tumors occurred in the ileum.

The earliest changes in the small intestine during carcinogenesis were mucosal hyperplasias. Later there was sometimes a rather rapid transition of small areas into infiltrating carcinoma which began with a loss of epithelial differentiation in the neck of the crypts and cessation of cell migration to the villi. Soon atypical crypt cells began to infiltrate the lamina propria. In agreement with the findings of SCHAUER *et al.* (1969) alkaline phosphatase activity in the brush border did not decrease earlier than in microcarcinoma.

The majority of small bowel tumors were more or less differentiated adenocarcinomas but mucus-producing and mixed carcinomas were also observed. Focal differentiation of Paneth cells occurred within adenocarcinomas as well as in anaplastic carcinomas.

In a few cases benign villous adenomas developed in the ileum. They showed maximal labelling in the upper mucosal areas near the surface and thus displayed the same proliferative activity as adenomas of the large intestine. Stalked adenomatous polyps did not occur in the small intestine.

Mucosal hyperplasias were also the earliest changes in experimental cancerization of the colon and rectum. These lesions were mainly localized on mucosal folds and were characterized by marked elongation of the crypts with increased cell proliferation but well preserved differentiation towards the mucosal surface.

Careful investigation of serial sections revealed small adenomatous areas within the hyperplastic mucosa. Here the majority of DNA-synthesizing cells were found near the surface. The lesions showed a fan-like expansion to the sides until typical polyps developed. Increasing vascularisation of the growing polyp caused splitting of the muscularis mucosae and, in connection with a distension of the mucosal fold bearing the polyp, stalk formation. Polyps with more than one proliferative center became lobulated.

The change in epithelial proliferation during polyp development was investigated quantitatively by evaluation of the ^{3}H-index in 5 mucosal zones between base and surface, in samples of normal and hyperplastic mucosa and in adenomatous polyps.

In normal mucosa the regeneration zone occupied about 60% of the mucosal thickness and the proliferative maximum was in the lower two zones. In hyperplasia the proliferation zone was extended to 80%, but normal conditions were maintained because the index maximum was still in the lower two zones and the superficial cells were differentiated. An essential quantitative change occurred in adenomatous polyps, where the proliferation zone was extended up to the mucosal surface and even the index maximum was transposed to a zone near the surface, i. e. at complete change from normal conditions had taken place. The results were statistically significant and confirmed our quantitative findings in human specimens (WIEBECKE, 1970; WIEBECKE *et al.*, 1969 a and b, 1970, 1973) as well as observations in hereditary polyposis of COLE and MCKALEN (1963) and DESCHNER *et al.* (1963).

The morphogenetic mechanisms of polyp development can be outlined as follows: An initial hyperplastic stage is succeeded by a partial loss of epithelial differentiation, so that proliferating cells shift up to the mucosal surface, where maximal epithelial proliferation is established. The result is a marked increase in tissue growth at this site which, by branching and twisting of gland tubes, causes a mainly horizontal expansion (WIEBECKE, 1970; WIEBECKE *et al.*, 1969 a and b, 1970, 1973) until typical fungiform polyps are developed.

In villous polyps, which because of their small number were not evaluated quantitatively, the index maximum was also transposed to the upper mucosa. Here we noted a vertical trend of growth but the factors inducing this different kind of growth are unknown.

The majority of tumors produced experimentally were broad based polyps with signs of malignant degeneration and polypous carcinomas. However, microcarcinomas without polypous precursors were found on several occasions as a result of rapid malignant transformation — the so-called "de novo-carcinomas".

Most of the neoplastic lesions seen in human intestinal mucosa could be reproduced experimentally by 1,2-dimethylhydrazine, which demonstrates that cancerization of the large intestine often runs a long course with development of polypous precursors. However a short course with rapid dedifferentiation and malignant transformation without visible precursory lesions is also possible.

References

COLE, J. W., MCKALEN, A.: Cancer (Philad.) **16,** 998 (1963).
DESCHNER, E., LEWIS, CH, M., LIPKIN, M.: J. clin. Invest. **42,** 1922 (1963).
DRUCKREY, H., PREUSSMANN, R., MATZKIES, F., IVANKOVIC, S.: Naturwissenschaften **53,** 557 (1967).
SCHAUER, A., VÖLLNAGEL, TH., WILDANGER, F.: Z. ges. exp. Med. **150,** 87 (1969).
WIEBECKE, B.: Habilitationsschrift Köln 1970.
WIEBECKE, B., LÖHRS, U., GIMMY, J., EDER, M.: Z. ges. exp. Med. **149,** 277 (1969 a).
WIEBECKE, B., LÖHRS, U., BRANDTS A., EDER, M.: Verh. Dtsch. Ges. Path. **53,** 239 (1969 b).
WIEBECKE, B., BRANDTS, A., EDER, M.: in preparation.
WIEBECKE, B., BRANDTS, A., LÖHRS, U., KREY, U., EDER, M.: 4th World Congress of Gastroenterology 1970, Copenhagen.

Tumor Induction in the Rat Kidney with Different Doses of DEN (Diethylnitrosamine): Frequency, Latency and Morphology of the Tumors

U. Mohr and J. Hilfrich

Introduction

In experimental animals, kidney tumors are induced by, among other chemicals, nitroso compounds. Tumors were found in rats after oral administration of dimethylnitrosamine [1, 7, 8, 10, 13] and also after oral, intravenous and intraperitoneal treatment with diethylnitrosamine [1, 2, 9, 12] or nitrosomethylurea [2, 6, 11]. Dose and duration of the carcinogen treatment influenced the frequency and the latent period of the kidney tumor. We have tested the carcinogenic effect of different single doses of diethylnitrosamine (DEN) in rats, and also sought to determine the smallest tumor-inducing dose as well as the single dose leading to a high percentage of kidney tumors.

Materials and Methods

Eighty male and 80 female, 3 months old Sprague-Dawley (WIGA) rats were used. The rats were divided into 8 groups and DEN was injected intravenously. The dose was 1.25 to 160 mg of DEN/kg body weight (geometric progression). The solvent saline was given to controls (10 males and 10 females) intravenously.

Animals were kept for life in Makrolon cages under standardized conditions (room temperature 22 ± 1° C, humidity 55 ± 5%, air change 8 times per hour, Hope Farms diet and water ad libitum). All the animals were autopsied. (One male control and one male from the 160 mg dose group were not evaluated because of cannibalism.) Organs were fixed in buffered formalin (4%) and embedded in paraffin. Eight sections of every kidney were stained with hematoxylin-eosin and van Gieson.

Results

The average survival of the animals is recorded in weeks (Fig. 1). As the carcinogen dose increased, survival decreased. Female rats lived an average of 6 weeks longer than the males. The survival of the low dose experimentals was longer than the controls (Fig. 1).

In the 120 weeks of the experiment no kidney tumors were observed in controls, either macroscopically or microscopically. In the experimental animals the tumor frequency was 5% for females and 3.8% for males up to the 60th week. After

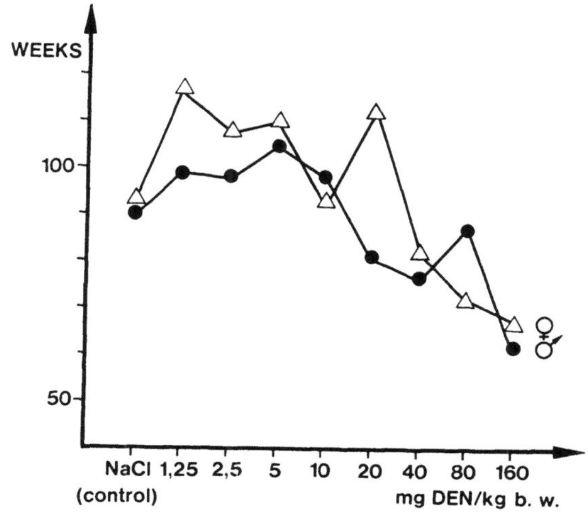

Fig. 1

120 weeks, 27.5% of the females and 17.7% of the males had neoplasms in the kidneys. Table 1 summarizes these results. The first tumor in the kidney was found in a female rat 41 weeks after treatment with 160 mg DEN/kg body weight. The first tumor in a male animal of this group was seen after 60 weeks. Rats which died before the 60th week after treatment showed single kidney neoplasms only in the dose groups 40—160 mg/kg body weight. After the 60th week the frequency of kidney tumors increased, also in the low dose groups. The smallest single dose of 1.25 mg DEN/kg body weight led to the development of a tubular kidney adenoma in a female rat 108 weeks after treatment. In groups with the high carcinogen doses more bilateral neoplasms of the kidney were seen than unilateral tumors and in female rats the frequency was higher than in males (Fig. 2).

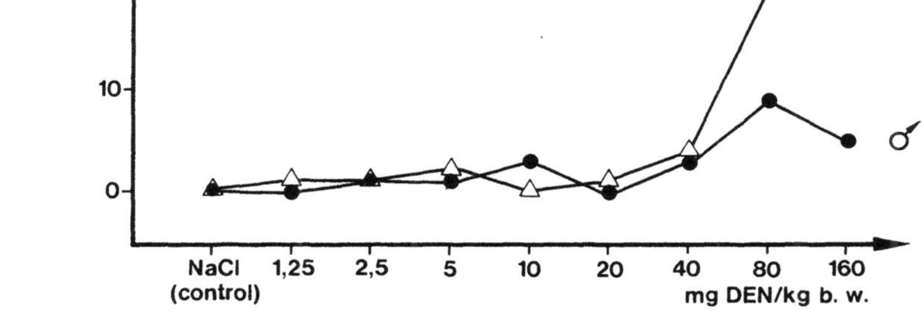

Fig. 2

Table 1. Patterns of kidney-tumors in Sprague-Dawley-rats after single intravenous treatment with DEN (mg/kg b. w.)

	Tumors up to 60 weeks						Tumors up to 120 weeks					
Dose	♂	uni-lateral	bi-lateral	♀	uni-lateral	bi-lateral	♂	uni-lateral	bi-lateral	♀	uni-lateral	bi-lateral
NaCl (Solvent)	0/9	—	—	0/10	—	—	0/9	—	—	0/10	—	—
1.25	0/10	—	—	0/10	—	—	0/10	—	—	1/10	1	—
2.5	0/10	—	—	0/10	—	—	1/10	1	—	1/10	1	—
5.0	0/10	—	—	0/10	—	—	1/10	1	—	2/10	2	—
10.0	0/10	—	—	0/10	—	—	3/10	3	—	0/10	—	—
20.0	0/10	—	—	0/10	—	—	0/10	—	—	1/10	1	—
40.0	2/10	2	—	0/10	—	—	3/10	3	—	3/10	2	1
80.0	0/10	—	—	1/10	1 [a]	—	3/10	—	3	6/10	1	5
160.0	1/9	—	1	3/10	—	3	3/9	1	2	8/10 [b]	1	7
Total	3/79 = 3.8%	2	1	4/80 = 5.0%	1	3	14/79 = 17.7%	9	5	22/80 = 27.5%	9	13

[a] malignant mesenchymal tumor

[b] one tubulary carcinoma with lung metastases

Histologically all of the kidney tumors were epithelial neoplasms except for 1 mesenchymal kidney tumor in a female rat treated with 80 mg DEN/kg body weight. This tumor was seen 44 weeks after treatment. In the first five groups (1.25 to 20 mg DEN/kg body weight), only benign kidney tumors were seen (adenomas) while the single intravenous injection of 40 mg DEN/kg led to a tubular adenocarcinoma in a female animal surviving 79 weeks. In the high dose groups (80 and 160 mg DEN/kg body weight), an increasing number of multiple, frequently bilateral carcinomas were seen, especially in female rats. Up to 4 tumors were found in one kidney (Fig. 3). The epithelial neoplasms developed only in the renal cortex and reached a maximum diameter of 5 cm (Fig. 4).

Microscopically, the epithelial tumors showed predominately expansive growth and were limited by pseudocapsules consisting of compressed kidney tissue (Fig. 5). Solid, tubular and cystic papillary patterns were seen with oxyphilic or oncocytic cells. Mitosis or nuclear polymorphism was rare. Variously extended necroses and single bleedings were frequent in the large tumors (Fig. 6). In the section of the mesenchymal sarcomatous kidney tumor, mainly spindle-shaped cells and numerous mitoses were found. In contrast to the epithelial neoplasms, tumor cells invaded the surrounding kidney parenchyma.

Metastases of tubular carcinomas of the kidney were found in one female rat treated with 160 mg DEN/kg body weight. After 91 weeks, extended lung metastases were found.

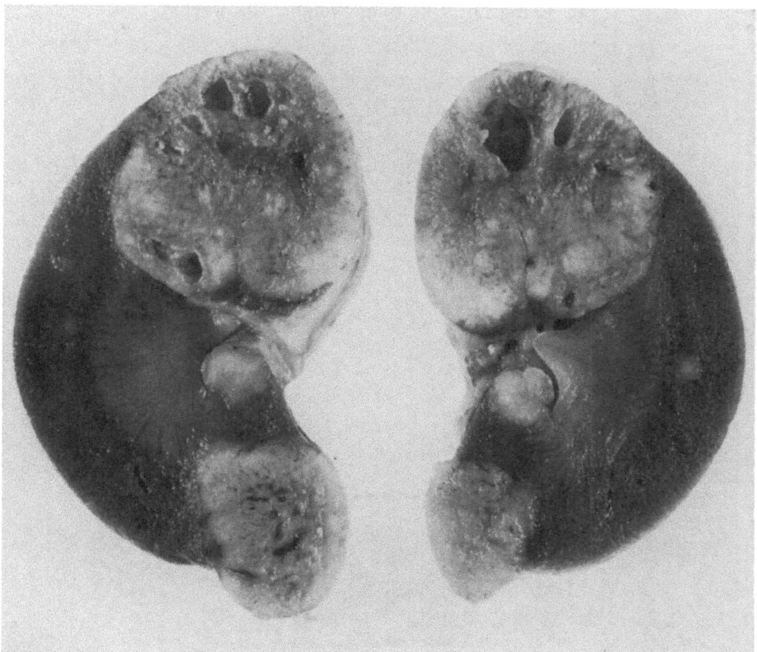

Fig. 3. Surface of kidney section with multiple epithelial tumors. Papillary cystic carcinomas in the upper and lower portion and different sized adenomas (female rat, 80 mg DEN/kg body weight, 116 weeks)

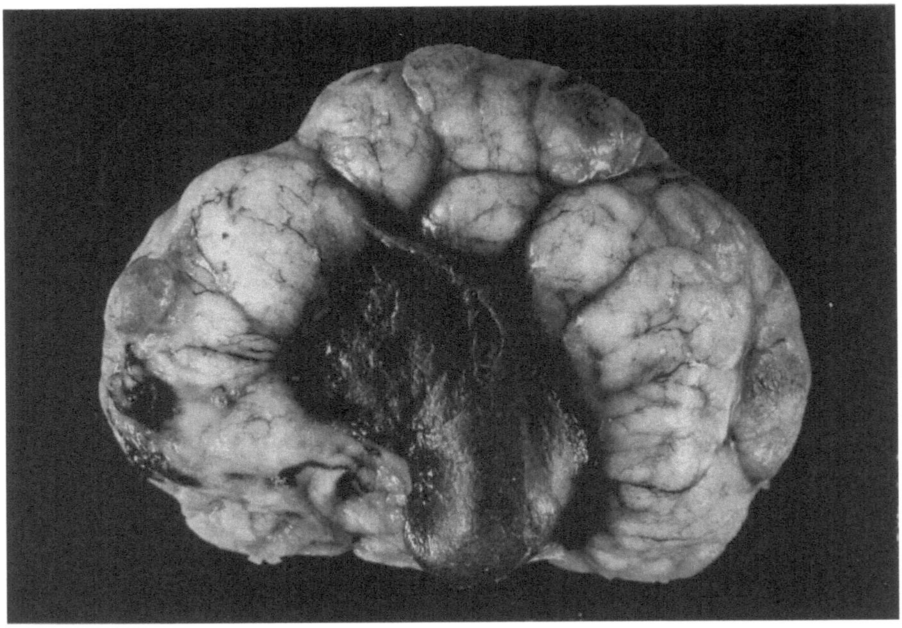

Fig. 4. Extensive tubular carcinoma with only a remaining small part of kidney tissue (female rat, 40 mg DEN/kg body weight, 108 weeks)

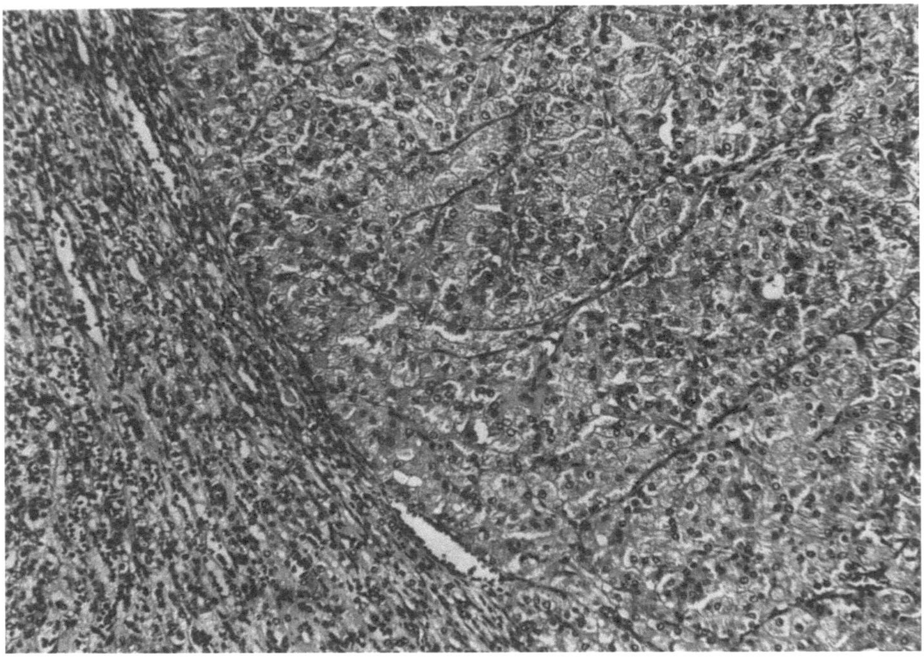

Fig. 5. Solid to tubular adenoma with mainly uniform cell patterns and pseudocapsule consisting of compressed kidney tissue. HE × 130

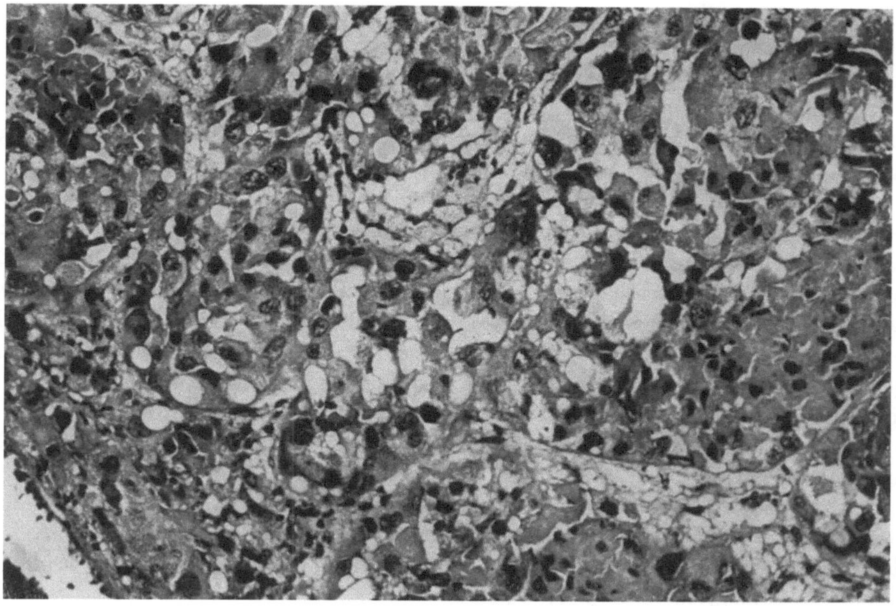

Fig. 6. Portion of a large tubular carcinoma with nuclear polymorphism and cell necroses. HE × 200

In addition to the kidney tumors, occasional hepatomas, hepatocellular carcinomas, mammary and lung neoplasms and tumors of the nasal cavities, as well as some thymomas and malignant lymphomas were found.

Discussion

While extended morphological studies of kidney neoplasms after treatment with different nitroso compounds have been reported, quantitative data concerning the relationship between tumor development and latency as a result of carcinogen dose are rarely described. Our experiments were especially concerned with the dose-effect relationship.

Since in controls no kidney neoplasms were observed and since rats very rarely show spontaneous tumors of this kind [12], one can interpret the results in this set of experiments to mean that kidney tumors developed due to the application of the carcinogen. The results show that a single intravenous dose of 1.25 mg DEN/kg body weight can induce kidney neoplasms in rats. Increasing the dose to 40 mg DEN/kg body weight or higher resulted in an increased number of malignant and bilateral kidney neoplasms. This was most prominent in female rats, along with a decrease in survival. The latent period decreased in some cases to less than 60 weeks.

With the exception of one mesenchymal tumor, comparable to that reported by Hard and Butler [3, 4, 5], a total of 36 animals showed epithelial kidney neoplasms (tubular adenomas and carcinomas). Estimating the degree of malignancy of epithelial kidney tumors is difficult [2, 12, 14] since intermediate forms are found in the progression from adenoma to carcinoma, therefore, they can only be diagnosed subjectively as benign or malignant. Typical signs of malignancy are seen only in a few cases of experimentally induced tumors. Usually the cytological patterns are uniform. Metastasis as proof of the diagnosis of carcinoma is only possible in a few cases.

Previous examinations reported by DRUCKREY *et al.* [2] and THOMAS and SCHMÄHL [12] have shown that intermittent oral application of high doses or the single intravenous application of the LD50 of DEN (280 mg/kg body weight) leads to kidney tumors within 41 to 45 weeks. Only epithelial neoplasms of the kidney (adenomas and carcinomas) were seen. MAGEE and BARNES [8] administered dimethylnitrosamine to rats in the diet (200 mg/kg diet) for one week, and kidney neoplasms were found 47—112 weeks later. Histologically the tumors were well-differentiated tubular neoplasms and anaplastic sarcomatous tumors of uncertain histogenesis.

DRUCKREY *et al.* [2] found kidney tumors in 45% of the rats treated with single intravenous injections of 70—100 mg nitrosomethylurea/kg body weight. Histologically these tumors were malignant mesenchymal tumors (sarcomas), and no epithelial neoplasm was found. Only females developed kidney tumors. LEAVER *et al.* [6] described sarcomatous neoplasms of the kidney after the single oral application of 90 mg nitrosomethylurea/kg body weight.

By comparing the reported results with the data from this set of experiments, it could be shown that different histologic tumor patterns developed after application of the described nitroso compounds. While dimethylnitrosamine induced epithelial tumors as well as anaplastic and sarcomatous neoplasms, diethylnitrosamine led mainly to the development of epithelial tumors, while nitrosomethylurea induced only sarcomatous tumors.

Summary

A single intravenous administration of 1.25—160 mg DEN/kg body weight (geometric progression) induced kidney tumors in male and female Sprague-Dawley rats. At doses of 40 mg DEN/kg body weight, increases in tumor frequency and number of carcinomas were seen, along with decreased survival. Female rats showed a higher tumor incidence than males. Epithelial tumors were observed (tubular adenomas and carcinomas); only one animal showed a malignant mesenchymal kidney neoplasm. Our results, and the results reported by other investigators, show that there is a relationship between the chemical structure of the applied nitroso compounds and the type of tumor induced in the kidney.

References

1. ARGUS, M. F., HOCH-LIGETI, C.: J. nat. Cancer Inst. **27**, 695 (1961).
2. DRUCKREY, H., STEINHOFF, D., PREUSSMANN, R., IVANKOVIC, S.: Z. Krebsforsch. **66**, 1 (1964).
3. HARD, G. C., BUTLER, W. H.: Cancer Res. **30**, 2796 (1970).
4. HARD, G. C., BUTLER, W. H.: Cancer Res. **30**, 2806 (1970).
5. HARD, G. C., BUTLER, W. H.: Cancer Res. **31**, 337 (1971).

6. Leaver, D. D., Swann, P. F., Magee, P. N.: Brit. J. Cancer **23**, 177 (1969).
7. Magee, P. N., Barnes, J. M.: Acta Un. int. Cancer **15**, 187 (1959).
8. Magee, P. N., Barnes, J. M.: J. Path. Bact. **84**, 19 (1962).
9. Rabes, H., Hartenstein, R., Gminder, J.: Naturwissenschaften **2**, 102 (1971).
10. Riopelle, J. L., Jasmin, G.: J. nat. Cancer Inst. **42**, 643 (1969).
11. Terracini, B., Testa, M. C.: Brit. J. Cancer **24**, 588 (1970).
12. Thomas, C., Schmähl, D.: Z. Krebsforsch. **66**, 125 (1964).
13. Zak, F. G., Holzner, J. H., Singer, E. J., Popper, H.: Cancer Res. **20**, 96 (1960).
14. Zollinger, H.-U.: Virchows Arch. path. Anat. **323**, 694 (1953).

Respiratory Infections and the Pathogenesis of Lung Cancer*

P. NETTESHEIM, H. SCHREIBER, D. A. CREASIA, and C. B. RICHTER **

1. Introduction

Epidemiological investigations of the past 15 to 20 years leave little doubt that tobacco smoke is the most important single factor in the etiology of lung cancer. Nevertheless, many questions concerning the pathogenesis of this neoplastic disease — the role of predisposing host and environmental factors and the possibility of synergistic or potentiating effects from combinations of various biological, chemical, and physical agents — are still unanswered (ROE and WALTERS, 1965; SAFFIOTTI, 1969). Some evidence for the interaction of etiological factors has been obtained in humans exposed to radon daughters and cigarette smoke (SACCOMANNO *et al.*, 1971) and to asbestos and cigarette smoke (SELIKOFF *et al.*, 1968).

The topic of our investigations — infectious (and inflammatory) agents as possible potentiating factors in carcinogenesis of the respiratory tract — has been actively debated for many years (for review see SPENCER, 1963; ROE and WALTERS, 1965; MCCLUNG, 1967; ECK *et al.*, 1969). Chronic bronchitis, influenza pneumonitis, interstitial pneumonia, and tuberculosis are all thought to be associated with a high risk of lung cancer in man. However, because of the conflicting results of numerous clinical and pathological case studies (e. g. MACKLIN and MACKLIN, 1940; RAEBURN and SPENCER, 1957; MEYER and LIEBOW, 1965; STAVRAKY, 1971), it is difficult to come to any firm conclusion regarding the role of inflammatory processes in the development of bronchogenic carcinoma. This uncertainty is reflected in the ambiguity with which the subject is discussed in several reviews on lung cancer etiology (ROE and WALTERS, 1965; ECK *et al.*, 1969); and two recent epidemiological studies (MCCLUNG, 1967; STAVRAKY, 1971) deny completely the existence of any compelling evidence for or against an association of lung cancer with pulmonary infection (or for that matter with any other "precursor disease"). It appears to us that one of the reasons for this confusion lies in the fact that tobacco smoke, the major etiological factor in pulmonary carcinogenesis, also interferes with the pulmonary defense systems against infectious agents (e. g. RYLANDER, 1968, 1969), making it difficult to single out the effect of respiratory infection in the pathogenesis of human bronchogenic carcinoma.

---

* Research jointly sponsored by the National Cancer Institute, and by the U. S. Atomic Energy Commission under contract with the Union Carbide Corporation.

** From the Carcinogenesis Program, Biology Division, Oak Ridge National Laboratory, Oak Ridge, Tennessee 37830, U. S. A.

That oncogenic as well as non-oncogenic viral agents can interact with chemical carcinogens to enhance neoplastic responses has been shown in several tumor systems (MARTIN *et al.*, 1961; DURAN-REYNALS, 1963), but only a few investigators have studied this phenomenon in the respiratory tract (KOTIN and WISELEY, 1963; KOTIN, 1966; LEUCHTENBERGER and LEUCHTENBERGER, 1965; HARRIS and NEGRONI, 1967; NETTESHEIM *et al.*, 1970, 1971, a, b), even though this organ system, because of its intimate contact with the environment, may receive frequent exposures to both viral and chemical agents.

In this presentation we review the main efforts currently being made in our laboratory to determine whether respiratory infections can act as co-factors in the pathogenesis of lung cancer. In discussing the various experiments, we have tried to include pertinent data from the literature. It should be mentioned at the outset that there is no single answer: the variables to be considered in these studies are simply too numerous. The type of carcinogen, carcinogen dose, type of exposure (single, repeated, or chronic), type of microbial agent, type of infection (chronic or acute), time relationship between carcinogen exposure and infection, and species differences (depending on which infectious disease model is to be tested with which lung tumor model) all are factors that influence the outcome of experiments of this type.

Rather than present a biased sample of results that might tend to support or negate a co-carcinogenic effect of respiratory infection, we discuss our current research as it relates to the topic, even though the findings are sometimes equivocal, or possibly contradictory. By taking this approach we can indicate many of the complexities facing the laboratory researcher who chooses to work in this area and, simultaneously, provide a framework of suggestive results that might give impetus to further experimentation.

We will first discuss modifications of the lung tumor response by respiratory infection and then describe our studies that are concerned with alteration of some host responses that might be important in the induction and progression of pulmonary neoplasms. A number of mechanisms by which infections might alter the respiratory tract tumor response are summarized in Table 1.

Table 1. Hypothetical co-factor effects of respiratory infection on pulmonary carcinogenesis

1. Disturbance of mucociliary clearance
2. Disturbance of alveolar clearance
3. Alteration of metabolic clearance
4. Destruction of protective cell layers
5. Disturbance of cellular steady state with increased cell proliferation (and faulty differentiation)
6. Suppression of immune surveillance mechanism

2. Effect of Respiratory Infection on the Lung Tumor Response Induced by Chemical Carcinogens

a) Influenza Pneumonitis

Between 1965 and 1970 we undertook a series of experiments designed to evaluate the carcinogenic and co-carcinogenic activity of various chemical, physical, and biological agents known or suspected to play a role in human lung cancer development (NETTESHEIM *et al.*, 1970, 1971 a, b). Three different air contaminants (ozonized gasoline fumes, Cr_2O_3 and $CaCrO_4$ particulates), X-irradiation, and PR8 influenza virus were used in these studies and were tested singly or in combination for tumorigenicity in the respiratory tract. The data will be reviewed here only insofar as they pertain to the interaction of respiratory infection and respiratory carcinogens.

Our investigation was prompted by the reports of KOTIN *et al.* (KOTIN and WISELEY, 1963; KOTIN, 1966; KOTIN *et al.*, 1958) describing the development of squamous cell tumors in the respiratory tract of C57BL mice exposed to ozonized gasoline fumes (synthetic smog) and three different respiratory viruses. One complication in these studies was the common occurrence of "spontaneous" pneumonitis in control animals (KOTIN *et al.*, 1958). Since one of our major objectives was to determine whether influenza pneumonitis would alter the tumor response to inhaled air contaminants (and X-irradiation), we conducted our experiments with mice free of respiratory disease. The mice were raised and maintained in a rigidly controlled barrier facility and were free of internal and external parasites, pathogenic bacteria, and eight common murine viruses (SIMMONS *et al.*, 1967). At 6 weeks of age, half of all the C57BL/6 mice used in the study were infected by aerosolization of lung homogenate containing influenza virus, strain PR8-34-60 (only animals positive for antiviral antibodies were used in the inhalation experiment). Two weeks later, daily exposure to one of three air pollutants was begun and was continued for the lifespan of the animal (5.5 hours per day, 5 days per week). We found that two of the air contaminants, synthetic smog and $CaCrO_4$ particles, caused a significant increase in lung tumor incidence. The effect of influenza virus infection on the lung tumor response induced by synthetic smog and $CaCrO_4$ exposure is illustrated in Fig. 1. A significant *reduction* in cumulative lung tumor incidence as well as a delay

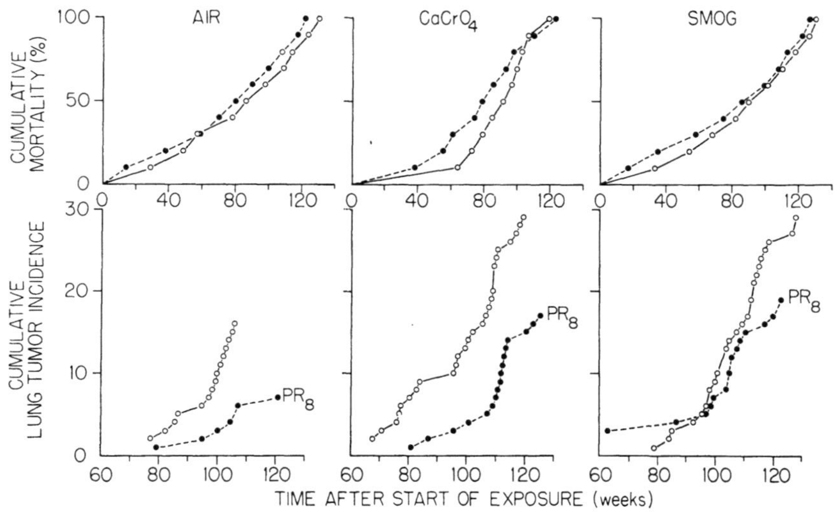

Fig. 1. Cumulative mortality and lung tumor incidence in C57BL/6 mice exposed to various air contaminants. ○, Uninfected mice; ●, mice infected with PR8 influenza virus

in the appearance of lung tumors was observed in the infected groups. Analysis of survival data showed that these differences were not the result of differences in mortality rates (NETTESHEIM *et al.*, 1970, 1971 b). Thus a true suppression of either tumor induction or tumor growth seemed to have occurred in the animals infected with influenza virus. All tumors were classified as pulmonary adenomas or adenocarcinomas. No squamous cell metaplasias or squamous cell tumors were observed.

Our finding of an inhibition of the pulmonary adenoma response in influenza-infected animals, though unexpected, is not unique. The first evidence for such a suppressive effect was suggested by CAMPBELL (1940), who exposed influenza virus-infected mice to dust containing coal tar and found a lower lung tumor incidence in the infected animals. Subsequently, STEINER and LOOSLI (1950) observed that influenza pneumonitis delayed the appearance of spontaneous pulmonary adenomas in strain A mice and resulted in a lower tumor incidence (compared with that of uninfected mice) in at least one of the two reported experiments. Though the authors were uncertain about the statistical significance of these findings, they felt that a "possible inhibitory or anticarcinogenic effect of influenza virus" might exist. In KOTIN's own study (1966), such an inhibition of the lung adenoma response is apparent (Table 2), since mice exposed to "flu-viruses" and to flu-viruses plus smog had a lower incidence of pulmonary adenomas than the corresponding control mice. The nature of this seemingly inhibitory effect of the influenza pneumonitis on the pulmonary adenoma development is presently unclear. One possible explanation is that it is due to the permanent loss of rather large amounts of alveolar parenchyma from pneumonitis and subsequent extensive fibrosis with complete atelectasis, frequently of one or two entire lung lobes. This explanation might particularly apply to situations where the tumors are expected to arise many months after the infectious episode. Studies are presently underway in our laboratory to determine whether this inhibitory effect of the influenza pneumonia can also be demonstrated with the faster developing urethane-induced lung adenomas in BALB/c mice, and whether the time relationship between carcinogen exposure and viral infection is critical.

In contrast to KOTIN's findings (KOTIN and WISELEY, 1963; KOTIN *et al.*, 1958), squamous cell tumors did *not* occur in our studies. It is known that squamous metaplasias can develop in mice and rats suffering from chronic murine pneumonitis, and it has been pointed out repeatedly that lesions induced by infectious agents can, to some extent, resemble neoplastic lesions (WINTERNITZ *et al.*, 1920; LOOSLI, 1949; LEUCHTENBERGER and LEUCHTENBERGER, 1965; RICHTER, 1971). This seems to be

Table 2. Incidence of tumor-bearing animals [a]

	No. of C57BL mice	No. of Survivors	No. of tumor-bearing animals	
			Pulmonary adenoma	Squamous cell carcinoma
Control	450	330	28	0
Smog	450	231	45	0
Flu	450	270	17	0
Flu + Smog	450	328	16	33

[a] From KOTIN (1966).

particularly pronouced when exposure to toxic chemicals is superimposed on infection, as has been documented by LEUCHTENBERGER and LEUCHTENBERGER (1965), although these authors have not reported an augmentation of the lung tumor response in experiments in which tobacco smoke exposure and influenza virus infection were combined. Whatever the true nature of the lesions observed by KOTIN, we believe that the main reason for the discrepancies between his and our observations is the difference in the microbiological status of animals used.

Recently, STAEMMLER *et al.* (1970) reported induction of pulmonary carcinomas in mice 2—3 weeks after infection with PR8 influenza virus. Supposedly no other viral or chemical agent was involved that could account for this dramatic carcinogenic effect. However, in view of the extensive literature on experimental influenza virus infection, it is difficult to accept this claim until it has been convincingly demonstrated that the presumed tumors are truly invasive, metastasizing, or transplantable.

b) Chronic Murine Pneumonia

Chronic murine pneumonia (CMP) is common in many "conventional" mouse and rat colonies. The etiology and pathogenesis of this disease, as well as the problem it can create for the experimentalist whose animal colony is affected by it, have been discussed in two recent reviews (BRENNAN *et al.*, 1969; LINDSEY *et al.*, 1971). Histopathologically, the disease is characterized by bronchopneumonia, bronchiectasis, and abscess formation; metaplastic lesions in various parts of the respiratory tract are a common finding. The major etiological factor appears to be mycoplasma pulmonis, although other infectious agents may also play a role in the pathogenesis of the disease.

We decided to investigate the effect of this *chronic* respiratory infection, as a counterpart to *acute* influenza pneumonitis, on a rat lung tumor system (SCHREIBER *et al.*, 1972). The nitrosamine *N*-nitrosoheptamethyleneimine had been shown previously by LIJINSKY *et al.* (1969) to be highly carcinogenic for the respiratory tract and esophagus of rats. When it was given in the drinking water, squamous cell tumors developed in the lung within 25—30 weeks. This carcinogen-tumor system seemed to be particularly well suited to our purposes, since the nitrosamine will induce tumors in two organ systems while the infectious process involves only one of them. Thus, if the pneumonitis exerted an effect on the tumor response, we would know whether it was a systemic or a localized one.

Conventional Sprague-Dawley rats selected for clinical signs of respiratory illness were obtained from a commercial source. Shortly after their arrival in the laboratory, 29 of the rats were killed and autopsied to verify the pneumonia. Serological testing revealed serum antibodies against at least one of the respiratory viruses listed in Table 3; only 7 out of the 29 were negative for all three of the viral agents listed. *Mycoplasma pulmonis* could be isolated from 19 animals; and macroscopic lung lesions, indicative of CMP, were found in 24 of the 29 rats. Specific-pathogen-free (SPF) rats were used as controls. These animals were obtained from a colony originally derived (by Cesarian section) several years ago from the same commercial breeder stock that produced the infected animals. The diseased and SPF groups were housed in different isolation facilities but received identical treatment. The carcinogen was administered to the rats at night in the drinking water, at a concentration

Table 3. Evidence of preexisting and current respiratory infection in conventional Sprague-Dawley rats

Agent	No. positive / No. tested	(%)
Pneumonia virus of mice [a]	7/29	(24)
Sendai virus [a]	8/29	(28)
Respiratory corona virus [a]	15/29	(52)
Mycoplasma pulmonia isolates [b]	19/29	(66)
Gross lesions of chronic murine pneumonia at autopsy	24/29	(83)

[a] Serological results (Dr. JOHN C. PARKER, Microbiological Associates, Inc., Bethesda, Md.). Eighty-five rats were selected for experimentation on the basis of clinical signs of respiratory infection. Twenty-nine were killed for serological and bacteriological testing one week before the carcinogen treatment of the remaining rats was started.

[b] From upper and/or lower respiratory tract.

of 100 mg per 1000 ml of distilled water. The amount consumed was determined the following morning. The carcinogen administration was continued for 22 weeks. The calculated cumulative carcinogen dose per rat was 137—140 mg. Body weights were determined every 4—6 weeks (Fig. 2). No differences in body weights were observed between uninfected and infected animals of the same sex.

All animals were killed at 24 weeks after the start of the experiment. At autopsy the number and size of recognizable lung tumors were determined. (*N*-nitrosoheptamethyleneimine causes multifocal tumor nodules.) Abscesses and bronchiectatic lesions could be distinguished in almost all instances from lung tumor nodules, because the latter were firm and greyish white in color. All tumors were sectioned through their longest axis and processed for histology to verify the macroscopic diagnosis and, if necessary, to correct the gross tumor count. The rest of the lung tissue was sliced

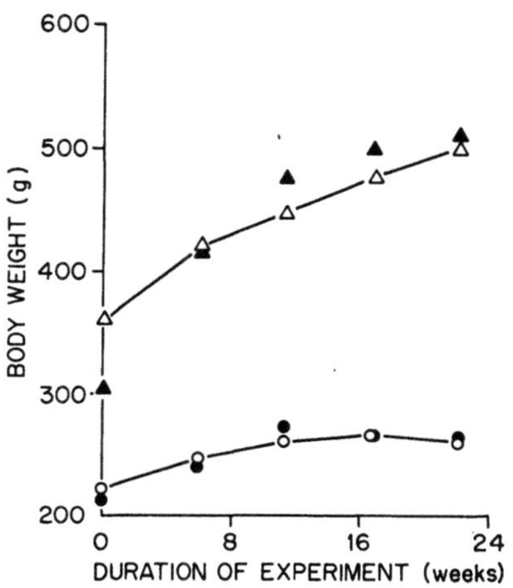

Fig. 2. Body weight changes in rats receiving *N*-nitrosoheptamethyleneimine in their drinking water. Male rats: △, SPF; ▲, with CMP. Female rats: ○, SPF; ●, with CMP. The rats were 10—12 weeks old at the start of the experiment

along the axis of the major bronchi and also processed for histology. Macroscopic and/or histologic evidence for murine pneumonia was obtained in all conventional but in none of the SPF rats treated with carcinogen. The tumor incidences in the various groups (after macroscopic and histologic evaluation) are summarized in Table 4. It can be seen that the number of animals with lung tumors is markedly higher in infected than in uninfected male rats. Similarly, the number of tumors per rat (or per tumor-bearing rat) is increased in infected males. In the female groups — which received a considerably higher carcinogen dose on a per gram body weight basis (because of the weight differences between the two sexes) — the difference between the uninfected and the infected groups ar not as striking, due to the fact that 19 out of 21 uninfected female rats had already developed tumors at the time of sacrifice. However, when the data are expressed as mean number of tumors per rat or per tumor-bearing rat, the infected females also had a significantly elevated tumor incidence. When the mean total tumor mass per rat lung was estimated, it was found to be 4 times greater in the infected than in the uninfected female rats (5200 mm³ as compared to 1100 mm³). No tumors were observed in infected control rats. In contrast to the lung tumor response, the esophageal tumor response was not altered by CMP. Histologically, all tumors, with the exception of a few microscopically visible adenomas (resembling the pulmonary adenomas in mice), were highly keratinizing squamous cell tumors. Neither the site of tumor development nor the morphological characteristics of the tumors appeared to be influenced by the infection. In addition to the lung tumors, massive squamous cell metaplasias were observed in the tracheobronchial tree of all carcinogen-treated animals (Fig. 3).

Our findings, though they have to be regarded as preliminary results and will need confirmation, strongly suggest that some respiratory infections may indeed significantly enhance the tumor response of the lung to chemical carcinogens. It should be pointed out that the present experiments were conducted under less than

Table 4. Lung tumor response to N-nitrosoheptamethyleneimine in specific-pathogen-free rats and rats with chronic murine pneumonia

Experimental groups	Effective no. of rats [a]	No. of rats bearing lung tumors [b]	Mean no. of tumors per rat	Mean no. of tumors per tumor-bearing rat	No. of rats with esophageal papillomas [b]
Specific-pathogen-free carcinogen-treated ♂	19 (21)	7 (37)	0.6	1.6	14 (74)
Chronic murine pneumonia carcinogen-treated ♂	29 (30)	24 (83)	2.8	3.4	22 (76)
Specific-pathogen-free carcinogen-treated ♀	21 (21)	19 (90)	2.5	2.8	17 (81)
Chronic murine pneumonia carcinogen-treated ♀	27 (30)	27 (100)	4.7	4.7	23 (85)
Chronic murine pneumonia untreated control ♀	25 (25)	0 (0)	—	—	0 (0)

[a] Only animals surviving entire carcinogen treatment were included in the study; numbers in parentheses indicate the number of rats at start of experiment.

[b] Numbers in parentheses indicate the percentage of tumor-bearing rats per group.

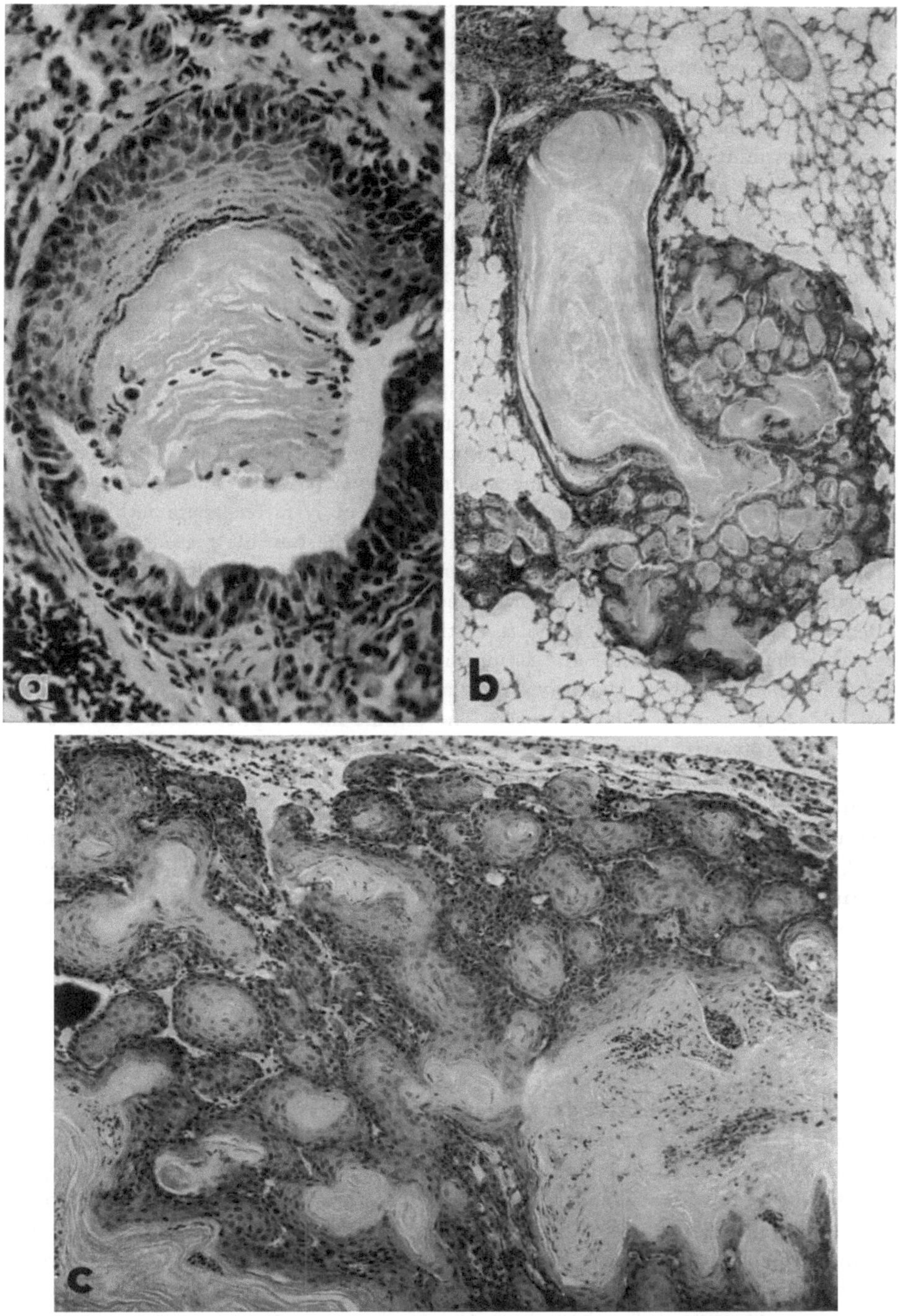

Fig. 3 a—c. Metaplastic and neoplastic lesions found in the respiratory tract of SPF and infected Sprague-Dawley rats after 22 weeks of *N*-nitrosoheptamethyleneimine administration in the drinking water. a Bronchus with keratinizing squamous metaplasia, b Keratinizing squamous cell lesion in bronchiole and peribronchiolar alveoli, c Squamous cell tumor occupying major part of a lung lobe ideal conditions, since the carcinogen dose applied was obviously too high to allow maximal expression of the enhancement effect. The mechanism underlying this enhancement of the lung tumor response to a "systemic" carcinogen is not known, but several possibilities are worth considering: increase of susceptible cell population or accelerated expansion of malignant clones due to increased cell proliferation (WARWICK, 1971) in the infected lung tissue; alteration of carcinogen metabolism in the infected lung; suppression of immunological surveillance by the heavy antigenic burden on the lymphatic tissues during the infection (microbial antigens).

The significance of our findings is potentially far-reaching, particularly since a great deal of attention is being given to the nitrosamines and nitrosamine precursors as potential carcinogenic hazards for man (e. g. LIJINSKY and EPSTEIN, 1970).

The two studies on the effects of respiratory infection on lung tumor responses presented here furnished seemingly contradictory results: influenza pneumonitis *suppressed* the pulmonary adenoma response in mice induced by carcinogenic air contaminants, while chronic murine pneumonia *enhanced* the squamous cell tumor response in the lung of rats developing as a result of *N*-nitrosoheptamethyleneimine ingestion. At present we can only speculate about the possible reasons for this discrepancy. Influenza virus inoculation causes an acute pneumonitis with extensive scarring and permanent obliteration of one or two lung lobes. Since the pulmonary adenoma is a tumor of the alveolar epithelium (type II alveolar cell), it is conceivable that the reason for the suppressive effect of the influenza pneumonitis is loss and/or modification (extensive alveolar metaplasia) of alveolar epithelium, i. e. loss of target tissue for the carcinogen. The chronic murine pneumonia, on the other hand, is a protracted inflammatory process, persisting for many months and involving all parts of the respiratory tract. It causes extensive hyperplasia and metaplasia, notably of the bronchial epithelium. Since the rat lung tumors induced by *N*-nitrosoheptamethyleneimine appear to be of bronchial (or bronchiolar) origin (LIJINSKY *et al.*, 1969), it is conceivable that the enhancement of this bronchial tumor response is caused by chronic regenerative and proliferative stimulation of the bronchial mucosa exerted by the persistent inflammatory process.

3. Alteration of Host Responses by Respiratory Infection

a) Pulmonary Clearance Mechanism

Tracheobronchial and alveolar clearance are probably the most important defense systems of the respiratory tract against inhaled toxic particles. The inhalation route is generally considered to be the main point of entry of environmental carcinogens into the respiratory tract, and it is believed that carcinogens entering by this route are usually in the form of particles or are carried by particles. Thus, factors disturbing pulmonary clearance are potentially of great importance as co-factors in carcinogenesis of the respiratory tract. A review of the current literature indicates that while extensive studies have been and are being conducted on the interference of inhaled noxious gases and particles with respiratory tract clearance, no systematic investigations on the disturbance of clearance by respiratory infection exists. The influenza virus infection appeared to be a good disease model with which to conduct the initial studies on this problem, since it destroys epithelium and produces inflammation both in the tracheobronchial tree and in the alveolar parenchyma (Fig. 6 a). (Thus it could be expected to interfere with the clearance mechanism on all levels of the respiratory tract.)

It also appeared advantageous that the influenza pneumonitis, in contrast to chronic murine pneumonia, is a rather acute disease, thus enabling us to study the recovery of impaired respiratory clearance as a function of time after the acute pneumonitic episode (CREASIA *et al.*, 1972 a, b).

Certain limitations are inherent in studies of respiratory clearance of radioactive particles in small rodents such as mice. Because of physical dimensions, it is difficult to distinguish with a nondestructive test between radioactivity located in various parts of the respiratory tract and in the upper digestive tract. After some initial exploratory studies using inhalation and intratracheal injection techniques with radioactive particles, we decided to use the latter method for particle deposition and whole-body counting as a means of determining the amount of radioactivity retained at various times after deposition. We recognized that this would introduce a certain artificiality into our experimental system, since intratracheally injected dust particles are mostly deposited in the deep lung, regardless of particle size. Therefore, information obtained with such a system will be largely confined to the lower respiratory tract clearance. The advantage is that whole-body counting can be used as a reliable measure of the lung burden, since alveolar clearance is so slow that no appreciable amounts of radioactivity are detectable in the intestinal tract at any given time other than the first 24—48 hours after intratracheal deposition. WATSON *et al.* (1969) recently demonstrated that the rate of particle clearance from the various pulmonary compartments is not appreciably different for inhaled or intratracheally deposited materials.

Specific-pathogen-free $BC3F_1$ mice were used in our study. Groups of mice were infected with influenza virus by intranasal inoculation. Only those animals positive for antiviral antibodies 2—3 weeks after inoculation were included in the study. Table 5 and Fig. 4 show the reproducibility of particle deposition and clearance in a large number of control mice. A total of 76 infected mice were used in the study. $^{51}Cr_2O_3$ was intratracheally administered either 2 days before, simultaneously with, or 1, 3, 5, 7, or 9 weeks after virus inoculation. In Fig. 5 the typical elimination patterns for animals with influenza infection are given; three experimental groups are included ($^{51}Cr_2O_3$ administration 2 days before, 1 week after, and 9 weeks after infection). It can be seen that the clearance of radioactive chromium was markedly

Table 5. Reproducibility of administering $^{51}Cr_2O_3$ to the lungs of mice by intratracheal injection

	Trial 1	Trial 2	Trial 3	Trial 4
No. of animals	10	10	10	10
Avg. dose [a]	279,136	274,357	254,373	255,112
Range	271,866 to 288,109	253,953 to 284,212	256,901 to 262,819	247,405 to 266,890
Standard error	± 1,545	± 2,665	± 809	± 1,594

[a] Counts/min, whole-body counting; 10.0 μg $^{51}Cr_2O_3$ approximates 2.5×10^5 counts/min.

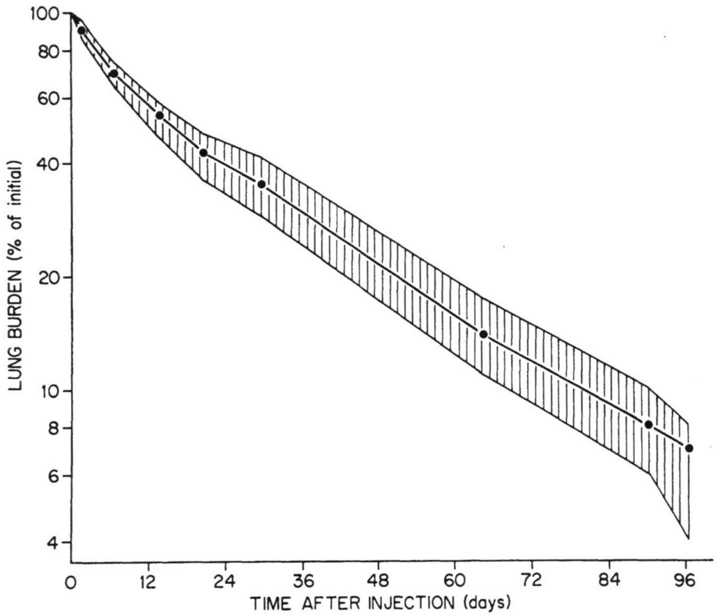

Fig. 4. Clearance of intratracheally administered $^{51}Cr_2O_3$ from the respiratory tract of uninfected mice. 10 µg of $^{51}Cr_2O_3$ (2.5×10^5 counts/min) were injected at time 0; whole-body counts were performed at various time intervals. Data are expressed as percentages of initial radioactivity remaining. Closed circles represent mean lung burden remaining (40 animals per time point); shaded area indicates range of values obtained

impaired in the majority of the animals in all three groups. At the end of the observation period, all animals were killed and were graded according to the amount of macroscopically discernible lung tissue scarring (consolidation and atelectasis). We found that all animals exhibiting impaired clearance showed massive consolidation and atelectasis of entire lobes, while animals with normal or near normal clearance had no grossly recognizable scarring of the lung tissue.

Histoautoradiograms prepared from the lungs of these mice revealed a significant difference in the localization of the radioactive dust particles dependent on the time of $^{51}Cr_2O_3$ administration relative to the time of virus inoculation. When the particles were administered before or simultaneously with virus inoculation, most of the radioactivity had aggregated in the consolidated lung lobes (Fig. 6 a—d). Presumably the radioactive chromium was deposited before the infectious process had taken hold and then was trapped in the inflamed and scarred tissues, which lose their connection to the rest of the bronchial tree. In the animals receiving $^{51}Cr_2O_3$ one or more weeks after the infection, the consolidated and heavily scarred tissue contained little radioactivity; instead, the lung lobes with only microscopic signs of a previous infection contained rather large amounts of radioactive material in thickened alveolar walls and small interstitial scars (Fig. 6 c). Thus the lung tissue only mildly involved in the infectious process sustained enough damage to exhibit a long-lasting defect of alveolar clearance.

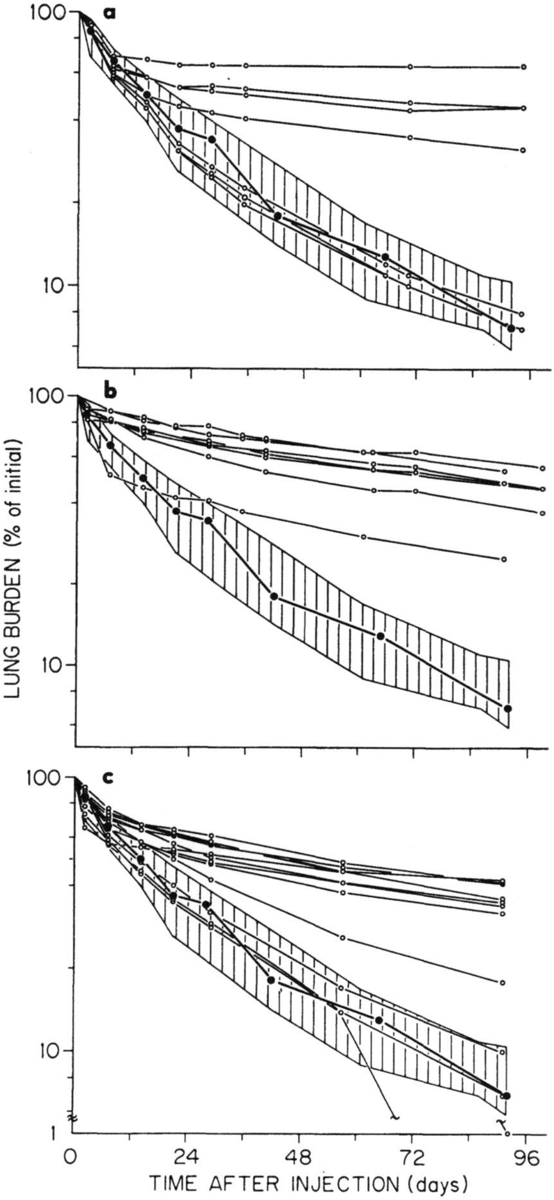

Fig. 5 a—c. Effect of influenza virus infection on $^{51}Cr_2O_3$ clearance from the respiratory tract of mice. 10 µg of $^{51}Cr_2O_3$ were administered intratracheally at different times before or after intranasal inoculation of PR8 influenza virus. Clearance in uninfected (●) and infected (○) mice was determined by whole-body counting. The control values are given as mean remaining lung burden calculated from 50 uninfected mice; shaded area indicates at various intervals. $^{51}Cr_2O_3$ was administered: a 2 days before inoculation with virus, high-low range. Data are expressed as percent of initially deposited radioactivity remaining, b 7 days after inoculation with virus, or c 9 weeks after inoculation with virus

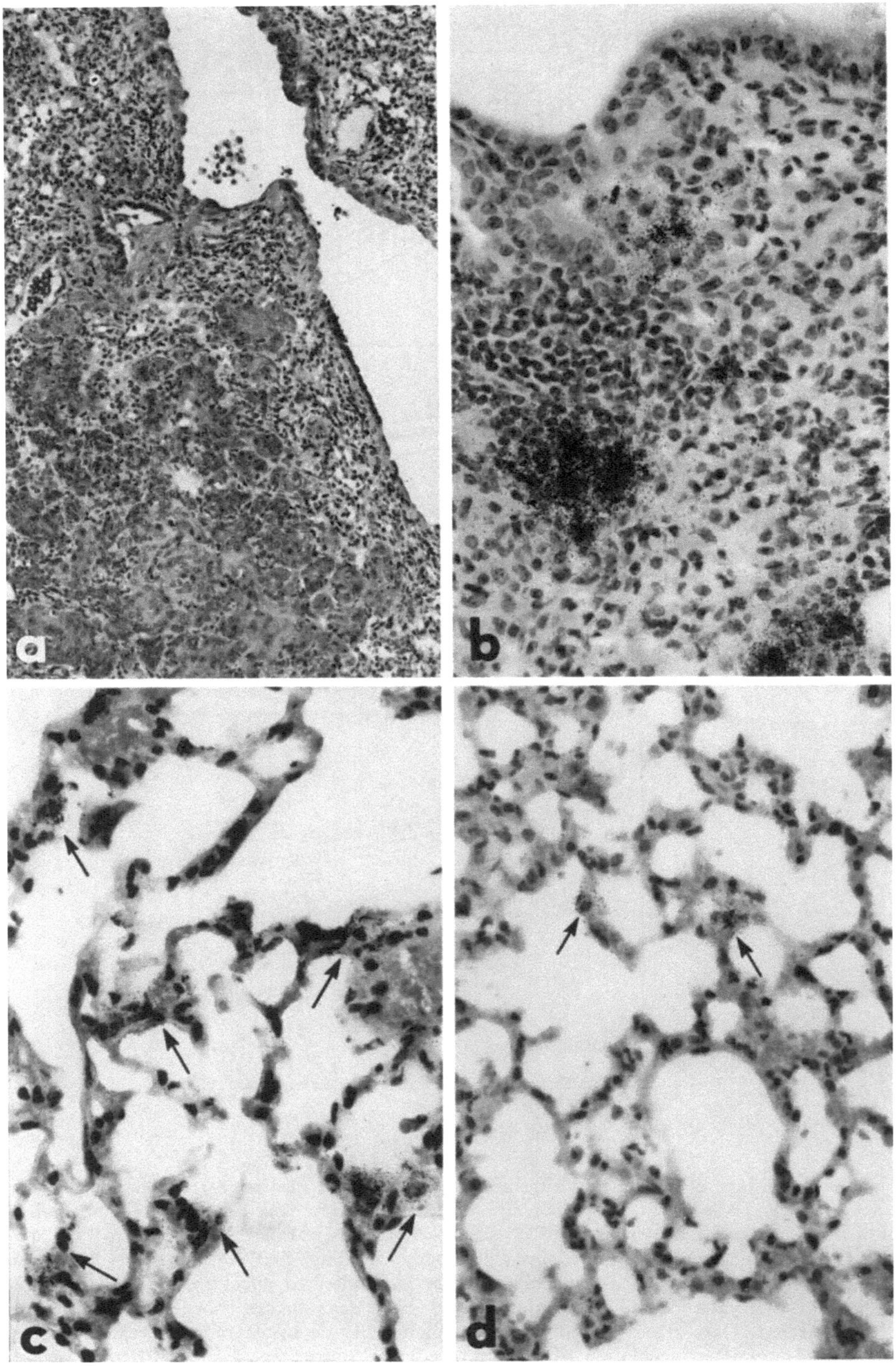
a
b
c
d

In summary, our experiments show that respiratory infections, particularly those that cause pneumonitis and subsequent scarring of alveolar parenchyma, can result in long-term impairment of pulmonary clearance. It does not seem unreasonable to assume that any other insult resulting in similar scarring and fibrosis of lung tissue (e. g. chemical insults, pulmonary embolism) will also cause comparable damage of the deep lung clearance.

Our findings may have serious implications for man, since the pulmonary residence time of radioactive particles may be considerably prolonged in damaged lung tissue, thus increasing the cumulative radiation dose. The fact that the dust particles aggregate in and near damaged lung tissue with formation of "hot spots" is probably also of significance, paraticularly in the case of radioactive particles, since the surrounding parenchyma will sustain a rather high radiation dose (see also Fig. 8 and 9 in NETTESHEIM *et al.*, 1971 a). Studies are presently underway to determine whether these results have a bearing on the pulmonary residence time of chemical carcinogens carried on dust particles.

b) Benzpyrene Hydroxylase Activity in the Lung

The capacity of tissues to metabolize chemical carcinogens to proximal carcinogens and also to less carcinogenic compounds (MILLER and MILLER, 1971), is an important factor in the overall carcinogenic process. It seems therefore important to determine whether factors such as microbial infections, which are being considered as co-carcinogens, influence the level and inducibility of enzyme systems involved in the metabolism of carcinogens (CORBETT and NETTESHEIM, 1973). Specific-pathogen-free BALB/c mice (female, 12—14 weeks old) were inoculated intranasally with a drop of a $10^{-7.0}$ dilution of a 10% lung homogenate containing PR8 influenza virus (which causes infection in 100% of the animals). In one series, mice were killed at 4, 7, and10 days after virus inoculation, and their benzpyrene hydroxylase activity was assayed according to the method described by NEBERT and GELBOIN (1968). Three to five mice were used per time point, with uninfected mice serving as controls. The results are summarized in Table 6. The enzyme activity found in infected lungs is expressed as a percentage of the enzyme activity obtained from lungs of control animals. It can be seen that the enzyme level becomes progressively lower as the

---

Fig. 6 a—d. Influenza pneumonia and its effect on $^{51}Cr_2O_3$ distribution and elimination. a Pneumonia 10 days after inoculation with virus; note loss of bronchial epithelium and consolidation of lung parenchyma with squamous-like metaplasia. (Hematoxylin and eosin; × 150.), b Autoradiogram from lung of mouse intratracheally inoculated with 10 μg of $^{51}Cr_2O_3$ 2 days before inoculation with virus. The animal was killed 90 days after injection of radioactive chromium. Note large aggregates of radioactive material in scarred lung tissue (compare with d). (Hematoxylin and eosin; × 375.), c Autoradiogram from lung of mouse intratracheally inoculated with 10 μg of $^{51}Cr_2O_3$ 3 weeks after inoculation with virus. The animal was killed 90 days after intratracheal injection of radioactive chromium. Large amounts of label are present in thickened and fibrosed alveolar walls of aerated lung lobe. (Hematoxylin and eosin; × 375.), d Autoradiogram from lung of uninfected mouse intratracheally inoculated with 10 μg of $^{51}Cr_2O_8$. The animal was killed 90 days after injection of radioactive chromium. Only small amounts of label can be detected in alveolar wall cells. (Hematoxylin and eosin; × 375.)

Table 6. Effect of influenza virus infection on benzpyrene hydroxylase levels in the lung [a]

Time	per mg of protein (% of control)	per total lung (% of control)
Day 4	84	88
Day 7	61	115
Day 10	12	20

[a] Measured in fluorometric units per 20 min incubation.

influenza pneumonitis develops. (The peak of the influenza virus lesion with maximum involvement of lung tissue is between 7 and 14 days.) These data indicate that besides physical clearance (see above) the metabolic clearance (and/or activation) is an important mechanism to be considered in studies concerned with the effect of respiratory infection on the lung tumor response to a polycyclic hydrocarbon.

c) Immune Response Elicited via the Respiratory Tract

It has been amply documented that the tumor response to viral and chemical carcinogens is often enhanced in immunologically suppressed animals and that transplantation of tumor cells is facilitated by immune suppression of the host (GOOD and FINSTAD, 1969; KLEIN, 1969; BURNET, 1970). The antigenicity of the tumor and the *overall immunocompetence* of the host are major factors which determine whether an effective immune response can be mounted against the developing tumor, or whether it will enhance tumor development (see PREHN, 1971, for discussion). There is evidence that *local lymphatic tissues* near the site of tumor origin respond to the antigens released by the tumor, although the significance of these lymph nodes in the host defense against the neoplasia is uncertain (BARD *et al.*, 1969; HAMMOND and ROLLEY, 1970; FISHER and FISHER, 1971). It is therefore important to determine the ability of these lymphatic tissues to respond to antigens, particularly since it is well known that the immune response is markedly influenced qualitatively as well as quantitatively by the route of entry of the antigen.

We decided to begin our investigation with one of the test antigens commonly used to study the humoral antibody response, namely, heterologous red blood cells (NETTESHEIM and WILLIAMS, in press). We found that antigenic stimulation via the respiratory tract is a very inefficient means of inducing a primary humoral immune response in comparison to intravenous (or intraperitoneal) antigen administration (Fig. 7a). A thousand times more antigen was required with intratracheal than with intravenous antigen injection to initiate a comparable antibody response in mice. In rats the differences between intratracheal and intravenous (or intraperitoneal) antigenic stimulation did not appear to be quite as great (Fig. 7b). The difference between the two species may be related to the greater amount of lymphatic tissue present in the lung proper of SPF rats. To obtain information regarding the site of antibody production following intratracheal antigenic stimulation of mice, we determined the number of hemolysin-forming cells in cell suspensions prepared from the lung, tracheobronchial lymph nodes, and the spleen, using the direct and indirect

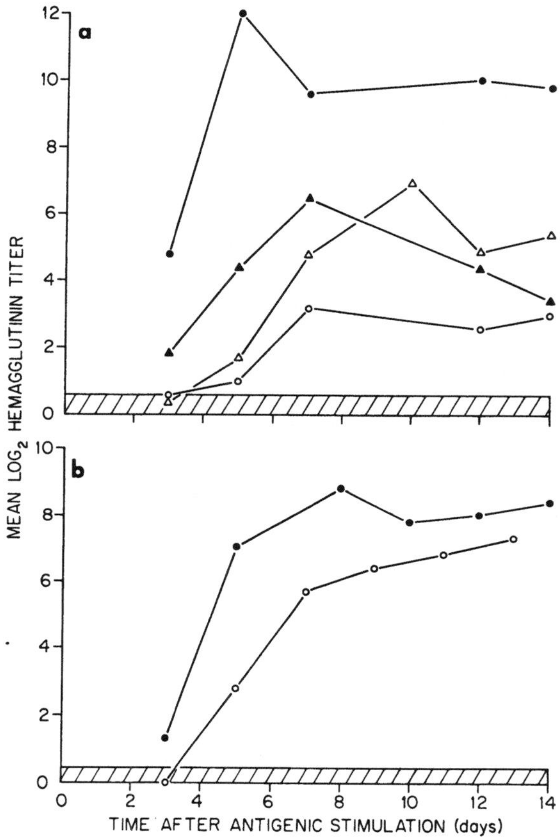

Fig. 7 a and b. Serum antibody response to sheep red blood cells (SRBC) in mice and rats. a BC3F$_1$ mice: 10^8 SRBC, intravenous (●); 10^8 SRBC, intratracheal (○); 10^9 SRBC, intratracheal (△); 10^6 SRBC, intravenous. ▲, b F-344 rats: 2×10^9 SRBC, intravenous (●); 2×10^9 SRBC, intratracheal (○). Five to ten animals per time point; shaded area indicates background titers

hemolytic plaque-forming assays as previously described (HANNA *et al.*, 1969). No more than 2—3% of the hemolysin-producing cells developing between 3—15 days in response to intratracheal injection of antigen were found in the lung and the lung-associated lymph nodes. Ninety-seven to 98% of the antibody-forming cells were found in the spleen (combined number of plaque-formers obtained from spleen, lung, and tracheal and bronchial lymph nodes were considered to be 100%). These data suggest that primary antigenic stimulation via the respiratory tract is very inefficient. At least in SPF mice and rats, the respiratory tract appears to be poorly equipped to respond to antigens. The major site of antibody production when elicited with massive antigen doses is *not* the respiratory tract and the associated lymph nodes but the spleen (we have not yet attempted to determine the gamma A antibody response after intratracheal administration of antigen).

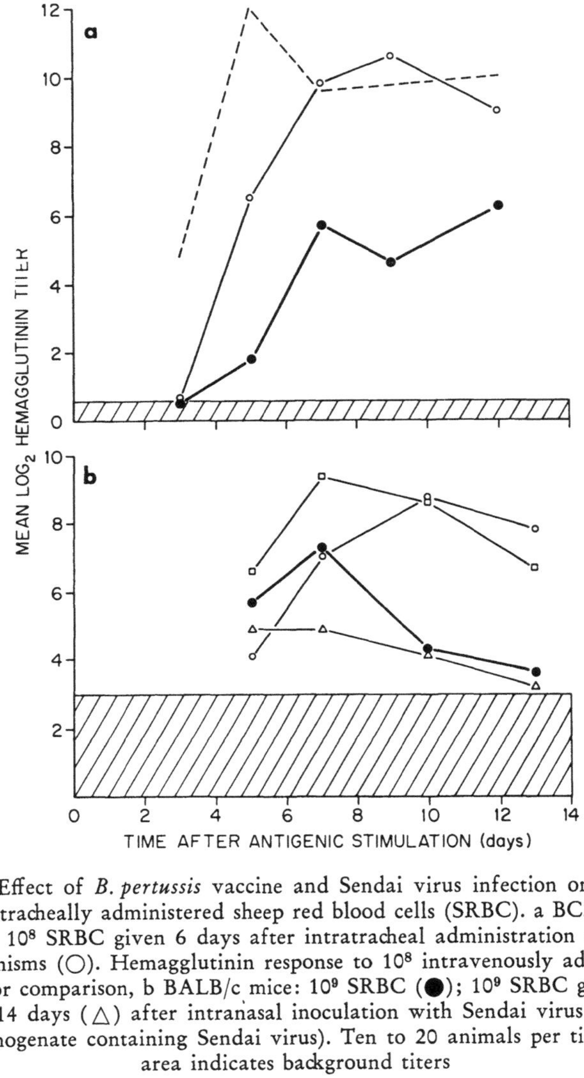

Fig. 8 a and b. Effect of *B. pertussis* vaccine and Sendai virus infection on serum antibody response to intratracheally administered sheep red blood cells (SRBC). a BC3F$_1$ mice: 5×10^8 SRBC (●); 5×10^8 SRBC given 6 days after intratracheal administration of 4×10^9 killed *B. pertussis* organisms (○). Hemagglutinin response to 10^8 intravenously administered SRBC (- - -) is given for comparison, b BALB/c mice: 10^9 SRBC (●); 10^9 SRBC given 4 days (○), 7 days (□), or 14 days (△) after intranasal inoculation with Sendai virus (10^{-3} dilution of a 10% lung homogenate containing Sendai virus). Ten to 20 animals per time point; shaded area indicates background titers

We then considered the possibility that this situation might change if the respiratory tract were exposed to bacterial or viral agents, since this often causes a severe influx of lymphoid elements into the lungs. Two studies were performed: one in which BC3F$_1$ mice were preexposed intratracheally to *Bordetella pertussis* vaccine, a potent adjuvant; and another in which BALB/c mice were preinfected with Sendai virus, a common respiratory tract pathogen in rodents. A marked enhancement of the antibody response was observed when the vaccine was given 1—14 days prior to stimulation with sheep red blood cells. Enhancement of the hemagglutinin response was maximal when the interval between vaccination and injection was 6 days (Fig. 8 a, b). The magnitude of the humoral antibody response under these conditions approximates that seen after intravenous administration of antigen. A study of plaque-forming ability showed that the number of hemolysin-forming cells in the lung and tracheobronchial lymph nodes was only twice that of mice not preexposed to *B. pertussis*. In contrast, the peak plaque-forming response in the spleen was approximately 20-fold greater in animals preexposed to *B. pertussis* than in those receiving only an intratracheal injection of sheep red blood cells. Thus, even in the vaccinated animal, the major organ producing antibodies to sheep red blood cells (gamma M and gamma G) is the spleen. Similar observations were made by KARELSE (1970) in a very extensive study, using tetanus toxoid as antigen.

The effect of Sendai virus infection on the hemagglutinin response to sheep red blood cells in BALB/c mice is summarized in Fig. 8b. It can be seen that an enhancement of the hemagglutinin response occurred during the first week of infection, and a suppression of immunocompetence occurred after the second week of infection, i. e. when sheep red blood cells were administered 14 days after intranasal inoculation with virus. (The results are somewhat complicated by the fact that BALB/c mice had rather high background titers.)

These experiments indicate that profound changes in the capacity to respond to antigens entering the respiratory tract can occur as a result of bacterial and viral infections of the lung. Further studies will be needed to determine whether the cell-mediated immune response, particularly against tumor antigens is similarly affected.

4. Summary and Conclusions

We have discussed the various experimental approaches currently being used in our laboratory to determine whether respiratory infection plays a decisive role in the pathogenesis of lung cancer. The tumor studies performed so far indicate that there is no single answer to the question: do respiratory infections enhance the lung tumor response to chemical carcinogens, and that the outcome of studies concerned with this problem will depend on the nature of the infectious disease (acute or chronic, major target site etc.) the carcinogen-tumor model (systemic or topical, acute or chronic exposure, target site etc.) and the time relationship between infectious and carcinogenic insult. One can only expect to determine whether and under what circumstances a particular respiratory infection will alter the neoplastic response of the lung in a given carcinogen animal model.

The few studies on *lung tumor response* and respiratory infection conducted to date can be summarized as follows: 1) In chronic inhalation studies performed with mice, influenza virus infection appears to suppress the pulmonary adenoma response induced by carcinogenic inhalants (NETTESHEIM *et al.*, 1970, 1971 a, b; KOTIN, 1966; CAMPBELL, 1940). 2) Development of squamous cell carcinomas was reported by KOTIN (1966) in mice exposed to synthetic smog and influenza viruses. 3) A significantly increased squamous cell lung tumor response to a cyclic nitrosamine was observed in rats suffering from chronic murine pneumonia (SCHREIBER *et al.*, 1972).

Investigations aimed at identification of *pathophysiological mechanisms* which might render the respiratory tract more susceptible to carcinogenic insults or might facilitate tumor development have also been described. Lung clearance studies showed that respiratory infection can significantly alter the distribution of inhaled (NETTESHEIM *et al.*, 1971 a) and intratracheally deposited (CREASIA *et al.*, 1972 a, b) particulates and can markedly increase the pulmonary residence time of particles deposited in the peripheral segments of the respiratory tract. These investigations also showed that recovery from this defect in deep lung clearance is very slow. At present, these studies have been performed only with PR8 influenza virus. Other microbial agents with an affinity for the respiratory tract will have to be tested in the future. It also needs to be determined whether these findings apply to chemical carcinogens (possibly adsorbed to carrier particles) deposited in the respiratory tract. Studies of the arylhydroxylase levels in the respiratory tract showed a marked alteration of benzo(a)pyrene metabolism during the course of influenza pneumonitis. Since the enzyme systems involved appear to be responsible for detoxification of the carcinogen as well as for the formation of the proximal carcinogen, it is presently difficult to decide what this suppression of the benzpyrene hydroxylase during infection means in terms of tumor induction.

Studies on the immune response elicited via the respiratory tract and its alteration by respiratory infection are presently limited to investigations of the humoral antibody response. The data indicate: 1) that there are considerable strain and species differences in the ability of rodents to respond to intratracheally injected antigens; 2) that the lung and lung-associated lymph nodes respond very poorly to antigens delivered to the respiratory tract, and that the main site of antibody production is the spleen; and 3) that exposure to *B. pertussis* or respiratory infection with Sendai virus markedly alters the antibody response to sheep red blood cells: an enhancement of the humoral antibody response occurred after stimulation with *B. pertussi* and during the first week after viral inoculation; a suppression of the antibody-forming capacity developed during the second week of the viral infection. The data indicate that it might indeed be very important to investigate thoroughly the changes in immunocompetence of the lung and lung-associated lymphatic tissues occurring during respiratory tract infection, since profound changes in the immunosurveillance against malignant tumors might occur in the cours of infectious respiratory disease.

We feel that our studies, even though they are still incomplete, have at this point yielded important information and have demonstrated the need for extensive experimental efforts to help resolve the old debate over the possible role of respiratory infection in the pathogenesis of lung cancer.

References

BARD, D. S., HAMMOND, W. G., PLICH, Y. H.: Cancer Res. **29**, 1379 (1969).
BRENNAN, P. C., FRITZ, T. E., FLYNN, R. J.: Lab. Anim. Care **19**, 360 (1969).
BURNET, F. M.: Progr. exp. Tumor Res. (Basel) **13**, 1 (1970).
CAMPBELL, J. A.: Lancet **1940 II**, 487.
CORBETT, T. H., NETTESHEIM, P.: J. Nat. Cancer Inst. **50**, 779 (1973).
CREASIA, D. A., NETTESHEIM, P., HAMMONS, A. S.: Hlth Phys. **23**, 865 (1972).
CREASIA, D. A., NETTESHEIM, P., HAMMONS, A. S.: Arch. environm. Hlth **26**, 197 (1973).
DURAN-REYNALS, M. L.: Progr. exp. Tumor Res. (Basel) **3**, 149 (1963).
ECK, H., HAUPT, R., ROTHE, G.: In: Handbuch der speziellen Pathologischen Anatomie und Histologie, III/4. Berlin: Springer-Verlag 1969, p. 250.
FISHER, B., FISHER, E. R.: Cancer (Philad.) **27**, 1001 (1971).
GOOD, R. A., FINSTAD, J.: Nat. Cancer Inst. Monogr. **31**, 41 (1969).
HAMMOND, W. G., ROLLEY, R. T.: Cancer (Philad.) **25**, 368 (1970).

HANNA, M. G., JR., NETTESHEIM, P., FRANCIS, M. W.: J. exp. Med. **129**, 953 (1969).
HARRIS, R. J. C., NEGRONI, G.: Brit. med. J. **4**, 637 (1967).
KARELSE, M. P. C.: Mechanismen van Respiratoire Immunisatie. Proefschrift. Rotterdam: Dukkerij Brouder-Offset N. V. 1970.
KLEIN, G.: Fed. Proc. **28**, 1739 (1969).
KOTIN, P.: In: Canadian Cancer Conference, Vol. 6. London: Pergamon Press 1966, p. 475.
KOTIN, P., WISELEY, D. V.: Progr. exp. Tumor Res. (Basel) **3**, 186 (1963).
KOTIN, P., FALK, H. L., MCCAMMON, C. J.: Cancer (Philad.) **11**, 473 (1958).
LEUCHTENBERGER, C., LEUCHTENBERGER, R.: In: Lung Tumours in Animals. Ed.: L. SEVERI. Perugia: Division of Cancer Research 1965, p. 445.
LIJINSKY, W., EPSTEIN, S. S.: Nature (Lond.) **225**, 21 (1970).
LIJINSKY, W. L., TOMATIS, L., WENYON, C. E. M.: Proc. Soc. exp. Biol. (N. Y.) **130**, 945 (1969).
LINDSEY, J. R., BAKER, H. J., OVERCASH, R. G., CASSELL, G. H., HUNT, C. E.: Amer. J. Path. **64**, 675 (1971).
LOOSLI, C. G.: J. infect. Dis. **84**, 153 (1949).
MACKLIN, M. T., MACKLIN, C. C.: Arch. Path. **30**, 924 (1940).
MARTIN, C. M., MAGNUSSON, S. M., GOSCIENSKI, P. J., HAUSER, G. F.: Science **134**, 1985 (1961).
MCCLUNG, J. P.: J. chron. Dis. **20**, 65 (1967).
MEYER, E. C., LIEBOW, A. A.: Cancer (Philad.) **18**, 322 (1965).
MILLER, J. A., MILLER, E. C.: J. nat. Cancer Inst. **47**, 5 (1971).
NEBERT, D. W., GELBOIN, H. V.: J. biol. Chem. **243**, 6242 (1968).
NETTESHEIM, P., HANNA, M. G., JR., DOHERTY, D. G., NEWELL, R. F., HELLMAN, A.: In: Inhalation Carcinogenesis. Oak Ridge: AEC Symposium Series No. 18, 1970.
NETTESHEIM, P., HANNA, M. G., JR., DOHERTY, D. G., NEWELL, R. F., HELLMAN, A.: In: Morphology of Experimental Respiratory Carcinogenesis. Oak Ridge: AEC Symposium Series No. 21, 1971.
NETTESHEIM, P., HANNA, M. G., JR., DOHERTY, D. G., NEWELL, R. F., HELLMAN, A.: J. nat. Cancer Inst. **47**, 1129 (1971).
NETTESHEIM, P., WILLIAMS, M. L.: Ann. N. Y. Acad. Sci., in press 1973.
PREHN, R. T.: Res. J. reticuloendothel. Soc. **10**, 1 (1971).
RAEBURN, C., SPENCER, H.: Brit. J. Dis. Chest **51**, 237 (1957).
RICHTER, C. B.: In: Morphology of Experimental Respiratory Carcinogenesis. Oak Ridge: AEC Symposium Series No. 21, 1971.
ROE, F. J. C., WALTERS, M. A.: Progr. exp. Tumor Res. (Basel) **6**, 127 (1965).
RYLANDER, R.: Acta physiol. scand. (suppl.) **306**, 1 (1968).
RYLANDER, R.: Arch. environm. Hlth **18**, 551 (1969).
SACCOMANNO, G., ARCHE, AUERBACH, O., KUSCHNER, M., SAUNDERS, R., KLEIN, M. G.: Cancer (Philad.) **27**, 515 (1971).
SAFFIOTTI, U.: Progr. exp. Tumor Res. (Basel) **11**, 302 (1969).
SCHREIBER, H., NETTESHEIM, P., LIJINSKY, W., RICHTER, C. B., WALBURG, H. E., JR.: J. nat. Cancer Inst. **49**, 1107 (1972).
SELIKOFF, T. J., HAMMOND, E. C., CHURG, J.: J. Amer. med. Ass. **204**, 106 (1968).
SIMMONS, M. L., RICHTER, C. B., FRANKLIN, J. A., TENNANT, R. W.: Proc. Soc. expt. Biol. (N. Y.) **126**, 830 (1967).
SPENCER, H.: London: Pergamon Press 1963, p. 623, p. 645.
STAEMMLER, M., FOITZIK, E., HEYDENREICH, M.: Z. Krebsforsch. **74**, 238 (1970).
STAVRAKY, K. M.: J. chron. Dis. **23**, 691 (1971).
STEINER, P. E., LOOSLI, C. G.: Cancer Res. **10**, 385 (1950).
WARWICK, G. P.: Fed. Proc. **30**, 6, 1760 (1971).
WATSON, J. A., SPRITZER, A. A., AULD, J. A., GUELTHOFF, M. A.: Arch. environm. Hlth **19**, 51 (1969).
WINTERNITZ, M. C., WATSON, J. M., MCNAMARA, F. P.: The Pathology of Influenza. New Haven: Yale University Press 1920.

Experimental Tumors of the Nervous System

Morphology and Morphogenesis

H. D. MENNEL

1. Introduction

The successful production of tumors of the nervous system by DRUCKREY *et al.* (1964) and IVANKOVIC *et al.* (1966) yielded a wealth of new data concerning the methods and results of such experiments. Although the molecular and cellular mechanism in the development of these neoplasms remain unknown, many new morphological and statistical facts could be collected. However, these morphological and statistical data need cautious analysis and interpretation. Only under this condition can useful conclusions for general pathology be drawn.

2. Morphology of Single Tumor Types

2.1 *Pituitary adenomas* in rats were observed during experimental tumor induction with neurotropic carcinogens (MENNEL, 1969).

The morphology of these blastomas was quite uniform. Single cells formed an homogenous layer and had the pale nuclei with clear nucleoli. No granula were visible after staining by the common methods used to differentiate pituitary cells. The more pleomorphic tissue architecture described earlier (MENNEL, 1969) proved to be exceptional as more material was accumulated.

2.2 *Olfactory neuroblastomas* were thought to be specific tumors of the posterior nasal cavity in hamsters and rats. Together with carcinomas they were observed when diethylnitrosamine (DEN) was given to hamsters (HERROLD, 1964) or certain cyclic nitrosamines to rats (DRUCKREY *et al.*, 1964). Such tumors were also produced with different substances of the azo-azoxyalkane-hydracin-group and with triacene derivatives.

In rats and hamsters, this tumor grows in the posterior nasal cavity and has a high tendency to invade and compress the forebrain. Small vascular septa are lined by a cylindrical epithelium, which sometimes copies the "medullary epithelium" by forming epithelial ribbons and hollow spaces. In other parts, true rosettes occur (Fig. 1).

2.3 *Sarcomas* of the brain and adjacent structures were induced in experimental animals by virus action (RABSON and KIRSCHSTEIN, 1960; VANDEPUTTE and BRUCHER, 1962) as well as through topical application of carbohydrates (ZIMMERMANN

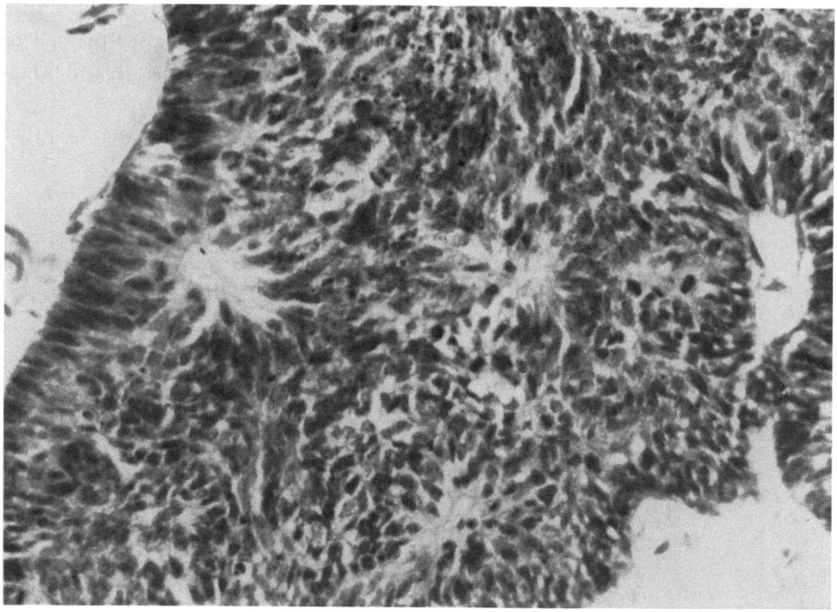

Fig. 1. Epithelial formations and rosettes are found in some tumors of the nasal cavity in small rodents. Note the occurrence of mitoses

and ARNOLD, 1943; SCHIEFER, 1958). In addition, some cerebral sarcomas were observed in rats (THOMAS and KERSTING, 1964) and in rabbits (JÄNISCH and SCHREIBER, 1967) during chronic experiments with methylnitrosourea (MNU).

All types of sarcomas (ZÜLCH and BINGAS, 1963) have been described for example fibrosarcomas of meninges (ZIMMERMANN and ARNOLD, 1943), spindle cell sarcomas (KAWAI, 1959), giant cell sarcomas (KAWAI, 1959) and reticulum cell sarcomas (SCHIEFER, 1958).

2.4 *Gliosarcomas,* i. e. mixed sarcomatous-gliogenic growth were observed in experiments with carcinogenic carbohydrates (SCHIEFER, 1962; PERESE and MOORE, 1960) and with nitrosamides, particularly, when MNU was applied to adult animals (JÄNISCH and SCHREIBER, 1967). SCHIEFER (1958) found islets of monster cells within true gliomas after administration of carcinogenic carbohydrates to mice. He observed, that the sarcomatous component of the tumor could originate from the capillary vessels of the new growth. KERSTING (1966) pointed out, that the sarcomatous part is usually located in the centre of the glioma.

2.5 *Gliomas, Ependymomas* and other groups of true neural blastomas were observed in a variety of experiments. In fact, all diagnoses were reported. This, however, is only partly due to different experimental conditions, the species of animals under investigation and to random distribution. The variation in diagnoses results also from the divergent use of nomenclature in classification. Our diagnoses are based on the work of ZÜLCH (1962) which comprises a classification and grading scheme. It was further elaborated by the rubrics of the UICC and gives room for some variables which are needed for the correct evaluation of growth characteristics (ZÜLCH and WECHSLER, 1968). This scheme has proved useful for classifying not only human but also experimental tumors (ZÜLCH and MENNEL, 1972).

Such a classification of experimental glial and paraglial tumors is given in Table 1. A short description of the single types follows.

Table 1. Classification of 833 gliomas and ependymomas experimentally induced in the brain. Tumors were observed in transplacental experiments with ethylnitrosourea, azoethane, ethylnitrosobiuret, azoxyethane and diethylhydrazine and in postnatal experiments with ethylnitrosourea in neyborn and young animals

Oligodendrogliomas	%
isomorphic	17,2
polymorphic	0,2
Astrocytomas	
isomorphic	10,4
polymorphic	0,4
Mixed gliomas	
isomorphic	36,4
polymorphic	8,2
Ependymomas	
isomorphic	24,5
polymorphic	2,7
	100,0

Oligodendrogliomas in rats have almost the same histology as in man. In solid tumors the classical honey-comb-architecture is seen. Simple augmentation of oligodendroglia cells between the fibres of the white substances or around nerve cells may be considered to be early stages of tumorous growth. Some large and even polymorphic blastomas of the oligodendroglia group may show totally or partly the same features (Fig. 2).

Astrocytomas in pure forms are less common (Fig. 3). Small neoplasms of this kind are often found in the subventricular tissue of the brain. This tissue is perhaps the origin of quite a number of experimental cerebral tumors.

Isomorphic mixed gliomas are composed of oligodendroglial and astrocytic cells. The mixture of these two cellular elements is so intimate, that the usual denomination "e potiori" is not possible. Apart from this the histological features are quite uniform.

Polymorphic gliomas, mostly polymorphic *mixed* gliomas, are so called because of their *cellular* or *tissular* variability. In the latter case, necroses (and occasionally other regressive changes), cellular proliferations (pseudopalisades) and newly formed vasculature are observed. Cellular polymorphism on the other hand is characterized by the varying size and shape of cells and the occurrence of giant cells (Fig. 4).

Ependymomas — isomorphic and polymorphic —, when they occur near the lateral ventricles, are slightly different from the forms typically seen in man such as those in the fourth ventricle and spinal cord (ZÜLCH, 1971). Therefore, we do

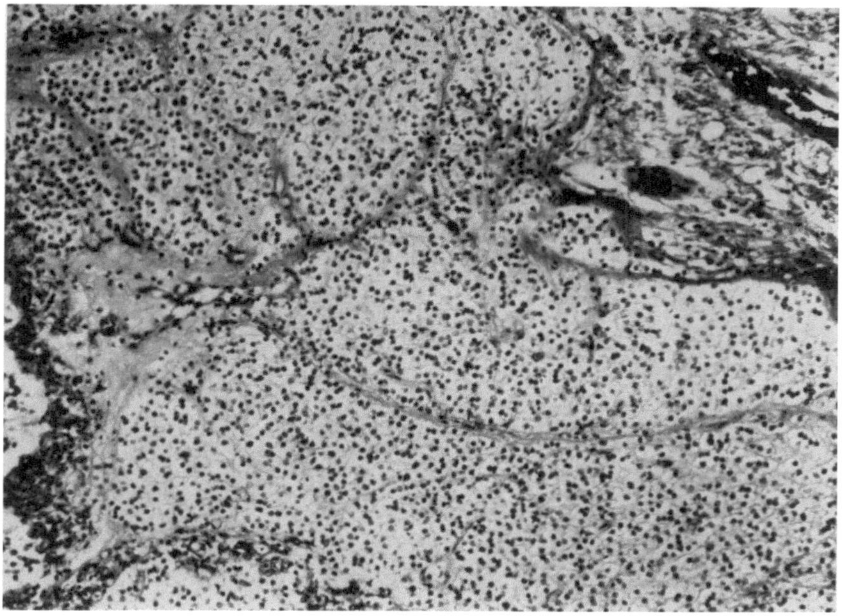

Fig. 2. Honeycomb formation of a middle-sized oligodendroglioma

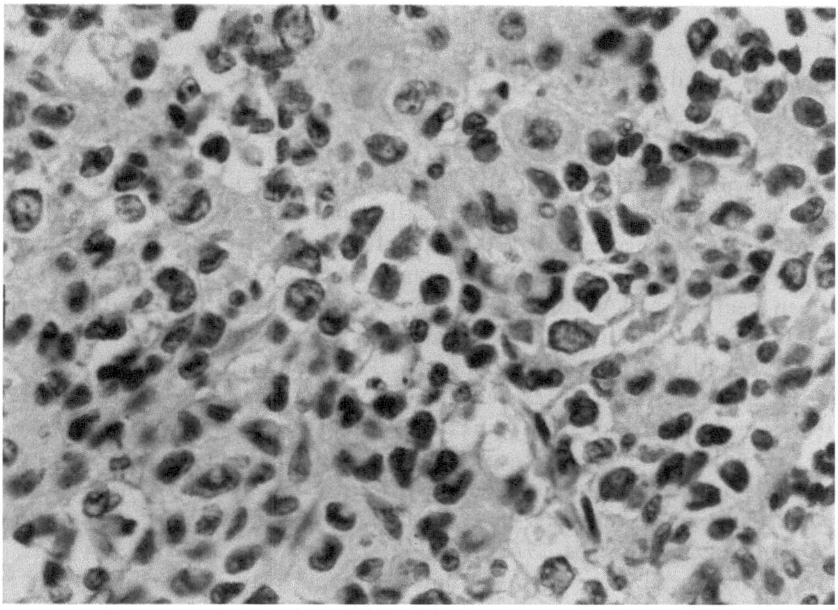

Fig. 3. The clear nuclei with fine, scarce chromatin in this tumors are considered to represent the astroglia of the brain. The more or less pronounced admixture of oligodendroglial cells is always visible

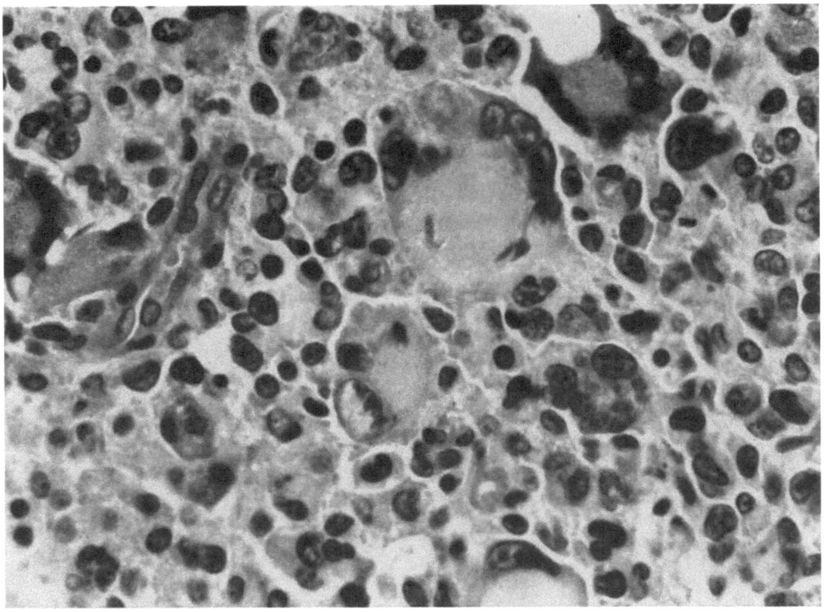

Fig. 4. These "Langhans-like" giant cells are interpreted by ZÜLCH as derived from the oligodendroglia. Their nature may be proved by impregnation techniques. In the experiments, this tumor type is rare

not always find the typical perivascular cuffs (Fig. 5). The most common feature of experimental ependymomas consists of short cellular columns within an unstructured ground substance.

2.6 *Nerve sheath tumors ("malignant neurinomas")* of experimental origin are rather frequent, but morphologically heterogeneous. Two types are prominent in these blastomas. One is the type with small round cells, comparable only to some forms of the human neurinomas. This type of tumor is rich in cells, but very often cyst formation is found. In the second type the fibrillary "streaming" architecture of human neurinomas (ANTONI, A) is represented. Neurofibroma — like fractions, which have very long streams of cells and are rich in collagen fibers are observed particularly in the peripheral small nerves. Lowly differentiated neurinomas again belong to different groups. In earlier publications, a separation of two or three different degrees of "differentiation" was used (WECHSLER *et al.*, 1969; KLEIHUES *et al.*, 1968). Depending on the occurrence or absence of reticulin fibers in these blastomas, sarcoma-like or medulloblastoma-like variants are distinguished. Yet it is not unusual for more than one of these tissue components to be seen in one single blastoma (Fig. 6), (MENNEL and ZÜLCH, 1971).

The general localization of these tumors is apparently in the nerve root. Some of them grow towards the spinal cord and produce neurological symptoms by compression. However, most of these tumors grow peripherally, following the path of the peripheral nerves, thus forming large cystic blastomas in the big plexuses or

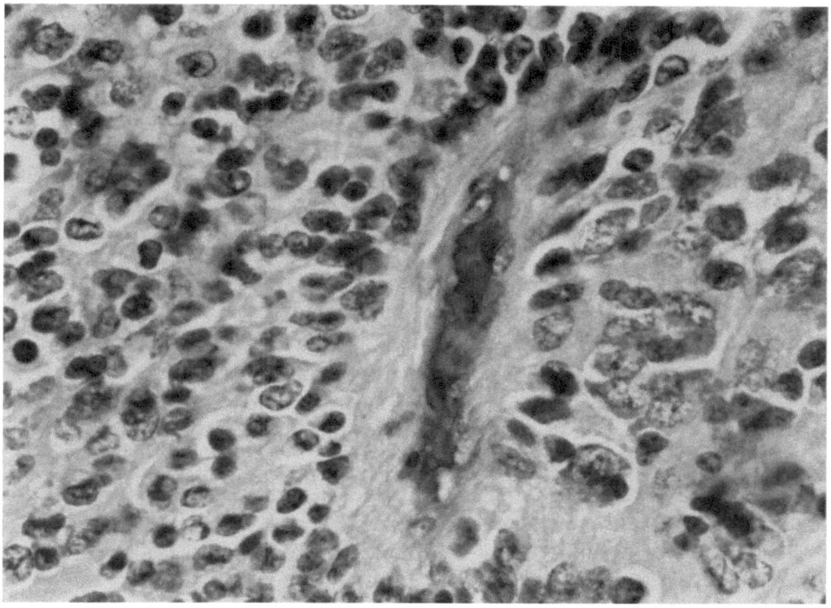

Fig. 5. Perivascular cuffs in an ependymoma of the rat

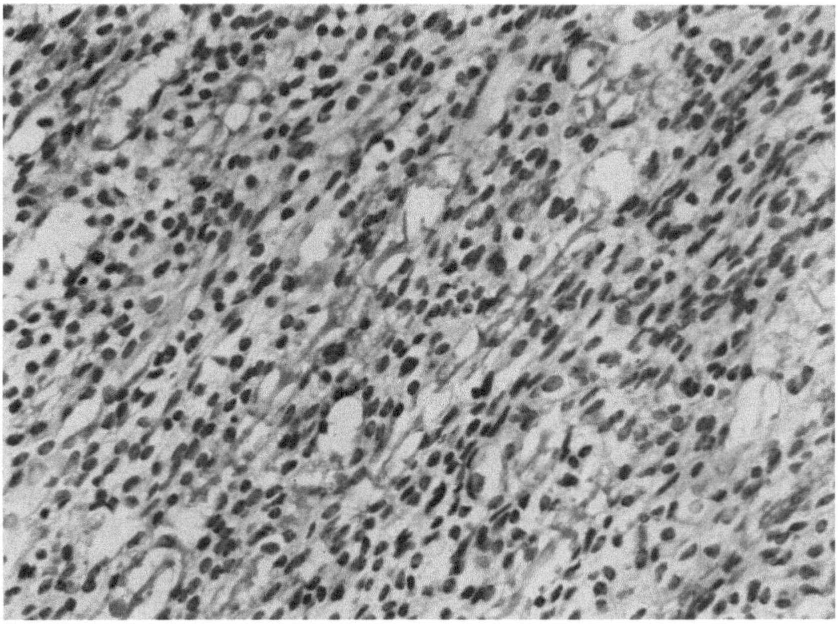

Fig. 6. The tumorous growth of peripheral nerve tumors follows the path of the nerve itself. Between the blastomatous cells, the generating myelin sheaths are visible

nerve trunks. The trigeminal is very often affected and here an infiltration of the root may stop at the zone where the brain tissue starts.

In hamsters, the transplacental action of ethylnitrosourea (ENU) led to another spectrum of resulting peripheral nerve tumors. Most of the tumors, which seemed to be less malignant, were situated in small nerves and had appearance of neurofibroma (MENNEL and ZÜLCH, 1972 a).

3. Aspects of Formal Pathogenesis

The obvious question arose, whether so-called spontaneous tumors of the nervous system may also be induced by exogenous factors. But it seems too early to give a comprehensive and final answer, but this may follow after extensive studies and accurate examination of the experimental conditions on the one hand and of statistical and biological data of human neurooncology, including particularly informative single cases on the other. This statement seems to be the neuropathologist's legitimate contribution to the "cancer problem" (ZÜLCH, 1969).

Both biological and morphological statistics of human nervous system tumors as well as the investigation of experimental tumor growth conditions have already been reported (ZÜLCH, 1956, 1971; ZÜLCH and WECHSLER, 1968; MENNEL and ZÜLCH, 1972 b). In this context, some special points relating to the experimental conditions producing the above mentioned morphological results will be described. These are: the influence of the *species* on the outcome, the role of *mesodermal* constituents in new growth of the nervous system, the *morphological* pecularities of intracerebral tumors and the *cytology* of Schwannomas.

3.1 The influence of the species seems most obvious in the occurrence of pituitary adenomas and olfactory neuroblastomas in rats.

Pituitary tumors in rats are probably dependent on hormonal activity. This view is supported by the fact that pituitary adenomas occurred almost exclusively in *old female* rats and that some of these animals had additional fibromas of the mammary gland. When these tumors were transplanted the grafted animals became unusually large (DRUCKREY and STEKAR, 1972). The cellular make up in genuine tumors and in grafted blastomas was rather uniform and similar to hyperplasias of mammo-somatotropic cells, which have to be considered as hormone dependent. Interestingly enough, subcutaneous transplantation into male and female rats also proved to be successful. The latency period of these transplanted tumors, however, was rather long. Up to now, the morphology in the first transplantation series did not change.

There are differences between the morphological pictures of pituitary adenomas in man and in rat and, as far as we can judge, in other species also (DONTENWILL, 1966). Therefore it seems noteworthy in this context that, apparently as a functional (hormonal) peculiarity of some species a predisposition to the formation of a certain tumor growth occurs, which although apparently hormone-dependent can also grow autonomously. No such behaviour is known to occur in adenomas of the human species.

The "*olfactory neuroblastomas*" are a good example of the role played by specific peculiarities of the local anatomy in experimental tumor formation. After the identification of these tumors as "esthesioneuroepitheliomas" in hamsters (HERROLD and DUNHAM, 1963) and in rats (THOMAS, 1965) the question arose, why this tumor, so extremely rare in man, could be produced regularly in these experiments. If the assumption (BERGERS, 1926) is correct that the tissue of origin of such blastomas is the olfactory mucosa, then it would be easy to understand that this tumor must be a rarity in man, whilst in *macrosomatic* animals it might occur more frequently.

3.2 In some cases definite problems arise in the diagnosis and classification of sarcomas, concerning the participation of mesodermal tissue in the formation of nervous system tumors, especially in the process of resorptive carcinogenesis. The frequency with which such tumors appear in experiments with local seeds of carcinogenic carbohydrates is perhaps due to the fact that the site of the pellet influences the tumor growth (SCHIEFER, 1958). When oncogenesis in the nervous system was induced with resorptive neurotropic carcinogens using *repeated* doses in *adult* animals, the proportion of sarcomas and mixed tumors of gliomatous-sarcomatous nature seemed to be always higher than in prenatal experiments and in tumor induction with *young* and *newborn* rats (ZÜLCH and MENNEL, 1970). However, even in chronic experiments with MNU in the rabbit, there are different interpretations about the participation of mesodermal constituents in brain tumors (JÄNISCH and SCHREIBER, 1967; KLEIHUES *et al.*, 1970), some probably identical tumors being classified as sarcomas by one and as polymorphic oligodendrogliomas by the other laboratory.

There seems to be a correlation between the participation of the mesoderm in tumor formation on the one hand and the size of the resulting tumors and the grade of polymorphism on the other (DRUCKREY *et al.*, 1972). This could be explained by the possibility that sarcomatous parts may originate from the vessel wall. Thus, glial-mesodermal mixed tumors are probably the consequence of the participation of the stroma in blastomatous growth.

3.3 Most data concerning the morphogenesis have been accumulated in the field of the genuine gliomas and ependymomas of the brain, especially during the last period of systemic tumor induction. The following general points must be discussed:

— multiplicity of tumor growth
— appearance of the early stages of tumor growth
— their point of origin and localization and
— cellular mixture and polymorphism of the resulting blastomas.

3.3.1 Multiple tumor growth in the central and/or peripheral nervous system is a common feature in experimental carcinogenesis with resorptive carcinogens. Tumors of the trigeminal nerve are found together with blastomas of central and peripheral nervous system. In the brain too, all stages of tumor growth may be seen. The number of tumors which occur however seems to depend upon the dose applied in the experiment, as shown by DRUCKREY *et al.* (1970) who gave single, variable doses of ENU to newborn and young rats. Similar results were obtained in transplacental experiments (IVANKOVIC and DRUCKREY, 1968).

3.3.2 The presence of tumors at *all stages* of growth permits the study of early forms of tumor formation, formerly named "microtumors" (WECHSLER *et al.*, 1969). They usually consist of minute clusters of cells in characteristic sites. They may occur as interstitial oligodendroglial cells, clusters of oligodendroglial cells around neurones, or by the multiplication of astrocytes in the subventricular glial zone. It is a constant feature that these early stages of tumor growth consist of pure cell population. During growth a change in cellular and tissular make-up of the tumor takes place.

3.3.3 Several observations indicate that the point of origin of most of the central nervous system tumors is the subventricular cell layer of the brain. Small blastomas are often found to be restricted to the subventricular cell layer, sometimes around the temporal horn, sometimes even growing symmetrically in both hemispheres. It is interesting to note that cell division still occurs in this region of the young, and even perhaps in the brain of the adult rat (Lewis, 1969). However, small blastomas may also occur in the white substance and even in the cortex of the experimental animals. Even in large blastomas a general arrangement around the ventricular system is obvious.

Further information about the actual origin of tumor growth in the brain may be gained by an analysis of the localization of brain tumors. The distribution of the different sites is given in Table 2.

Table 2. Localization of 833 gliomas and ependymomas experimentally induced in the brain in rats

White substance of hemisphere	32,3%
Ventricular system	23,1%
Subependymal region	12,1%
Hippocampus formation	7,6%
Brain stem	7,6%
Brain cortex	4,3%
Other localizations	12,9%
	99,9%

3.3.4 Although a mixture of glial cells is often seen in middle-sized tumors of the glioma group, cellular and tissular signs of polymorphism are only found regularly when the tumors are large and extend over a whole hemisphere. In this case an architectural mixture occurs and "oligodendroglial border zones" are found around "centrally" rather pure ependymomas.

Pure early forms of tumor growth of ependymomas are rare. Single examples of small epdendymomas and evidence of proliferative areas in the ventricular epdendym of the rat brain, however, may prove that these tumors in fact originate from the ventricular wall (Kleihues, 1972).

With regard to the cellular polymorphism one rather interesting point should be mentioned. In chronic experiments with MNU in rats as well as in rabbits tumors with giant multinucleated cells occurred. These "Langhans-like" cells behave as oligodendrocytes when impregnated by specific silver techniques. These tumors correspond well to be polymorphic oligodendroglioma in man described by Zülch, 1964. Other investigators have named the same tumor glioblastoma multiforme (Jänisch and Schreiber, 1969).

Since the degree of polymorphism seemed to be positively correlated with the size of the tumor, we attempted to determine whether this too could be dependent on the dose applied. In one instance this was apparently the case (Zülch and Mennel, 1972 b). This problem, however, needs further study.

3.4 Cytological criteria are decisive for the diagnosis of "malignancy", for instance of a neurinoma in the process of tumor formation. But correct identification of the cell of origin is difficult, when anaplasia in tumor growth occurs. Therefore attempts were made to identify the single cells within the tumor ensemble. Electron microscopy was used to differentiate Schwann's cells from fibroblasts in malignant neurinomas. Some authors have found that features characteristic of Schwann's cells were only identified in *some* of the tumor cells (Wechsler *et al.*, 1969; Georgson *et al.*, 1969). Here again it was not possible to decide whether this was due to cellular mixture or to loss of differentiation.

Almost the same observation has been made in transplantation and explantation experiments. Tumors of the trigeminal and spinal root were transplanted subcutaneously. Several generations after the transplants cells with the characteristics of Schwann's cells could still be identified in addition to fibroblasts. Both cell-types were able to migrate from the explant and to form large networks on the surface of the glass (Mennel, 1972).

The identification of these two cellular elements, the specific neurotropic action of the compounds used in the experiments and the similarity of this type of experimentally induced malignant neurinoma with the similar rather rare tumor in man (Mennel and Zülch, 1971) led to the hypothesis of the Schwannian origin of this tumor. This was despite the fact, that the morphology may change slightly in different species and under varying experimental conditions.

4. General Conclusions

In addition to the known results of topical application of carcinogenic carbohydrates, systemic doses of viruses and especially of chemical carcinogens have been used to induce nervous system tumors. The most surprising observation was the transplacental action of some of these substances. Of course, one may speculate that these models are also valid for the so-called spontaneous tumors in animals and in man. This problem has recently been discussed by Zülch (1969, 1971).

Without going into the details of the controversy, some statements can be made:

1. The nervous system may be considered a suitable subject for the discussion of exogenous tumor induction.

2. Although evidence of external causes of nervous system tumors in man is still lacking, preventative measures have to be taken to eliminate any dangerous substances from the human environment.

3. There is an urgent need to investigate further the role of carcinogenic chemical substances and viruses.

Summary

Experimental tumors of nervous origin are in some aspects morphologically similar to corresponding human neoplasms. In this case, conclusions as to the pathogenesis of neoplasms in human neurooncology are legitimate. On the other hand, considerable differences exist in some tumors between experimental and human new growth. These differences can only be partially explained by the experimental conditions and properties of the species under investigation. The general significance of experimental tumor production in the central nervous system has to be considered in the light of these findings with some reservation.

References

BERGER, L., COUTARD, H.: Bull. Ass. franç. Cancer **15**, 404 (1926).
DONTENWILL, W.: In: Handbuch der experimentellen Pharmakologie, Bd. 16. Erzeugung von Krankheitszuständen durch das Experiment, Teil 3, Tumoren II. Berlin-Heidelberg-New York: Springer 1966.
DRUCKREY, H., IVANKOVIC, S., MENNEL, H. D., PREUSSMANN, R.: Z. Krebsforsch. **66**, 138 (1964).
DRUCKREY, H., SCHAGEN, B., IVANKOVIC, S.: Z. Krebsforsch. **74**, 141 (1970).
DRUCKREY, H., STEKAR, J.: Personal communication 1972.
DRUCKREY, H., PREUSSMANN, R., IVANKOVIC, S., ZÜLCH, K. J., MENNEL, H. D: The experimental Biology of Brain Tumors. Eds. W. KIRSCH, P. PAOLETTI and E. GROSSI-PAOLETTI. Springfield: Charles C. Thomas Publ. 1972.
GEORGSSON, G., WESSEL, W., THOMAS, C.: Z. Krebsforsch. **72**, 12 (1969).
HERROLD, K. M., DUNHAM, L. J.: Cancer Res. **23**, 773 (1963).
HERROLD, K. M.: Cancer (Philad.) **17**, 114 (1964).
IVANKOVIC, S., DRUCKREY, H., PREUSSMANN, R.: Naturwissenschaften **53**, 410 (1966).
IVANKOVIC, S., DRUCKREY, H.: Z. Krebsforsch. **71**, 320 (1968).
JÄNISCH, W., SCHREIBER, D.: Naturwissenschaften **34**, 171 (1967).
JÄNISCH, W., SCHREIBER, D.: Experimentelle Geschwülste des Zentralnervensystems. Jena: VEB Gustav Fischer Verlag 1969.
KAWAI, S.: Acta path. jap. suppl. **9**, 707 (1959).
KERSTING, G.: Wien. klin. Wschr. **78**, 260 (1966).
KLEIHUES, P., MATSUMOTO, K., WECHSLER, W., ZÜLCH, K. J.: Verh. dtsch. Ges. Path. **52**, 672 (1968).
KLEIHUES, P., ZÜLCH, K. J., MATSUMOTO, S., RADKE, U.: Z. Neurol. **198**, 65 (1970).
KLEIHUES, P.: Personal communication 1972.
LEWIS, P. D.: Nature (Lond.) **217**, 974 (1969).
MENNEL, H. D.: Arzneimittelforsch. **19**, 1055 (1969).
MENNEL, H. D.: Z. Neurol. **201**, 269 (1972).
MENNEL, H. D., ZÜLCH, K. J.: Zbl. Neurochir. **32**, 11 (1971).
MENNEL, H. D., ZÜLCH, K. J.: Acta neuropath. (Berl.) **21**, 194 (1972 a).
MENNEL, H. D., ZÜLCH, K. J.: Acta neuropath. (Berl.) **21**, 140 (1972 b).
PERESE, D. M., MOORE, G. E.: J. Neurosurg. **17**, 677 (1960).
RABSON, A. S., KIRSCHSTEIN, R. L.: Arch. Path. **69**, 663 (1960).
SCHIEFER, B.: Zbl. Neurochir. **18**, 360 (1958).
SCHIEFER, B.: Acta Neuropath. Suppl. **I**, 19 (1962).
THOMAS, C., KERSTING, G.: Naturwissenschaften **51**, 144 (1964).
THOMAS, C.: Z. Krebsforsch. **67**, 1 (1965).
VANDEPUTTE, M., BRUCHER, J. M.: Acta neuropath. (Berl.) **1**, 397 (1962).
WECHSLER, W., KLEIHUES, P., MATSUMOTO, S., ZÜLCH, K. J., IVANKOVIC, S., PREUSSMANN, R., DRUCKREY, H.: Ann. N. Y. Acad. Sci. **159**, 360 (1969).
ZIMMERMANN, H. M., ARNOLD, H.: J. Neuropath. exp. Neurol. **2**, 416 (1943).
ZÜLCH, K. J.: In: Handbuch für Neurochirurgie, Bd. XII. Berlin-Göttingen-Heidelberg: Springer 1956.
ZÜLCH, K. J.: In: Classification of brain tumors. Wien: Springer 1964.
ZÜLCH, K. J.: Acta neurochir. (Wien) **10**, 639 (1962).
ZÜLCH, K. J.: Arzneimittel-Forsch. **19**, 1503 (1969).

ZÜLCH, K. J.: Atlas of the histology of brain tumors. Berlin-Heidelberg-New York: Springer 1971.
ZÜLCH, K. J., BINGAS, B.: Rev. brasil. Chirurg. **54,** 234 (1963).
ZÜLCH, K. J., MENNEL, H. D.: Proceedings of VI. Int. Congr. of Neuropath. Paris. Book of the Congress. Paris: Masson 1970.
ZÜLCH, K. J., MENNEL, H. D.: Zbl. Neurochir. **32,** 225 (1971).
ZÜLCH, K. J., MENNEL, H. D.: In: Handbook of clinical Neurology; Vol. 16, Tumors of the Nervous System (in press).
ZÜLCH, K. J., MENNEL, H. D.: Proceedings of the meeting of transplacental carcinogenesis. Hann. 1971. "Transplacental Carcinogenesis". IARC Scientific Publications No. 4. IARC Lyon 1973.
ZÜLCH, K. J., WECHSLER, W.: In: Progr. neurol. Surg. **2,** 1 (1968). Basel: Karger; New York: Year Book.

Tumor Organotropy of N-nitrosomethylurea under the Influence of Hormonal Contraceptives

C. THOMAS *

In recent years the oral contraceptives have been under discussion as tumor-inducing, or at least as potential carcinogenic agents. These hormones have been commercially available for oven ten years in West Germany, and have been used by over two million women. An increased cancer mortality or cancer morbidity has not yet been confirmed in this group. It is a well-known fact of human pathology, however, that the induction period of a tumor may well stretch out over decades, and thus the present negative findings do not yet have decisive significance. We are thus confined to animal experiments as a means of assessing possible carcinogenic effects. Until now these experiments have proved largely negative, and the potentiation of carcinogens by these contraceptives has also not been demonstrated. Never theless, there is a broad spectrum of viewpoints regarding the possible risk of cancer through the use of hormonal contraceptives. I call the reader's attention here to the contributions of DALLENBACH-HELLWEG (1969), OBER (1966), HILLEMANNS (1971) and others, which have been reported in part in the popular press.

Hormonal contraceptives are a combination of estrogenic and gestagenic hormones. Which observations from human pathology or from animal experiments allow us to rule out possible carcinogenic effects of the oral contraceptives or its components?

Progesterone has been causally associated with tumor induction by only a few authors. It is accepted that chlormandinone acetate and medroxyprogesterone acetate induce benign mammary tumors in female beagles. These tumors were demonstrated in five out of sixty female beagles subjected to long-term progesterone treatment at ten to twenty-five times the usual dose. Although these experiments clearly imposed exceptional conditions, these hormonal contraceptives were taken off market in the interest of caution.

Estrogens have been under discussion for years as carcinogenic agents, and uterine and mammary carcinomas especially have been regarded as estrogen-induced. It is well known from *human pathology* that hyperestrogenism can induce a glandular-cystic, and occasionally even an adenomatous hyperplasia of the uterus. The latter is considered to be precancerous. Mammary carcinomas have also been observed among men receiving long-term estrogen treatment for prostate carcinoma. On the other hand, WILSON (1962) reported that in 304 women treated with estrogen for

* Supported by the Deutsche Forschungsgemeinschaft, Bonn-Bad Godesberg.

osteoporosis or climacteric complaints for an average of 7,8 years, there by exposing the uteri and mammary gland to a total of 2387 patient-years, not a single, although 18 mammary or uterine neoplasms were statistically expected in this group, tumor was encountered (WALLACH and HENNEMANN, 1959, GORDAN, 1961). *Experimentally*, estrogen enrichment leads, in most cases, to neoplastic changes only in genetically predisposed animals, for example, mammary carcinomas in mice. Rhesus monkeys treated with estrogens for over seven years developed neither mammary carcinomas nor mammary precancer (GESCHICKTER and HARTMANN, 1959).

Hormonal contraceptives: No increase in the overall tumor rate especially not in mammary or uterine neoplasms is observed among women subject to long-term use of oral contraceptives. PINCUS (1961) did in fact demonstrate a decrease of nodular growth in the breast under ENOVID® treatment. In addition, there are no known cases which could be unquestionably and directly attributed to hormonal contraceptives. Malignant changes in portio dysplasias or carcinomata *in situ* were not observed following 5,5 years treatment with ENOVID®. Corresponding animal experiments have similarly proved largely negative.

It was also necessary to test whether the enrichment of hormonal contraceptives could influence the tumor-inducing action of a carcinogen. STERN and MICKEY (1959) established that the growth of dimethylbenzanthrene-induced mammary tumors in rats was inhibited by ENOVID®. Similar investigations were undertaken and similar results obtained in other organs and other species. The questions of whether an oral contraceptive can shift the organotropic effect of a carcinogen and whether tumors of other organs might appear more frequently than usual still remain. We have tested this question in animal experiments using nitrosomethylurea, which gives rise to a broad spectrum of organ tumors and the action of which is well known from previous studies (DRUCKREY *et al.*, 1967; THOMAS and BOLLMANN, 1969). One hundred and twenty, 140 g Wistar rats were employed in the experiment. Nitrosomethylurea (NMU), dissolved in water and adjusted to pH 4 with citrate buffer, was administered orally on three successive days at doses of 40 mg NMU/kg body weight. An aqueous suspension of 0,0075 mg mestranol and 0,25 mg lynestrenol, i. e. 1/10 of a tablet of 2,5 LYNDIOL® animal day was administered to rats in the experimental design is presented below:

1. NMU Control Group

Forty rats received 40 mg NMU/kg body weight by oral administration on three successive days.

2. NMU + OC Experimental Group

Forty rats received 40 mg NMU/kg body weight by oral administration on three successive days. Following a 30 day pause, the animals were treated with oral contraceptives (OC) for 30 days.

3. OC + NMU Experimental Group

Forty rats received oral contraceptives for 30 days followed by the carcinogen on the 31st, 32nd and 33rd experimental days.

Numerous tumors appeared in both control and experimental animals following NMU treatment, as shown in Table 1.

Esophageal papillomas and esophageal carcinomas can be accounted for by local action of the carcinogen, whereas the remaining neoplasms arose resorptively. Statistical evaluation of induction times shows no significant difference between control and experimental groups. On the other hand, the tumor yield, especially the number of nephroblastomas, is significantly decreased in the OC+NMU experimental group. However, the shortening or lengthening of induction times of the nephroblastomas could not be demonstrated.

The distribution of organ tumors in the NMU control group and the NMU+OC experimental group corresponds with the results of previous investigation (THOMAS and BOLLMANN, 1969). In addition, no macroscopic or histologic deviations were demonstrated among the esophageal and kidney tumors (THOMAS and SCHMÄHL, 1964; THOMAS and SO, 1969). It is noteworthy, however, that neither mammary nor uterine tumors developed in the experimental group pretreated with hormonal contraceptives.

These investigations support the views existing in the literature, insofar as we were unable to demonstrate any essential deviations in the organotropic effect of nitrosomethylurea as a result of prior or subsequent treatment with oral contraceptives. The only demonstrable difference was that rats pretreated with ovulatory

Table 1. Localisation and induction time (t_{50}) of tumors induced by nitrosomethylurea (NMU) before and after administration of hormonal contraceptives (OC)

Tumor	NMU	t_{50}	NMU+OC	t_{50}	OC+NMU	t_{50}
Nephroblastoma	18	285±56	14	258±41	7	269±65
Forestomach: carcinoma	6	247	11	257	5	260
Leukemia	7	268	4	229	6	187
Breast: carcinoma	3	225	4	241	0	—
Malignant thymoma	1	200	3	198	4	254
Malignant neurinoma	3	360	4	281	0	—
Glandular stomach: carcinoma	2	289	1	416	1	271
Uterus: sarcoma	1	230	0	—	0	—
Uterus: carcinoma	0	—	1	256	0	—
Mediastinum: sarcoma	0	—	1	232	0	—
Tongue: carcinoma	0	—	0	—	1	271
Glioblastoma multiforme	0	—	1	232	0	—
Malignant odontoma	0	—	1	220	1	206
Malignant tumors	41		45		25	
Breast: fibroadenoma	5	288	1	226	1	416
Lung: adenoma	0	—	2	192	0	—
Jaw: cholesteatoma	1	230	0	—	0	—
Kidney: cholesteatoma	0	—	1	277	0	—
Lipoma	0	—	0	—	1	271
Benign tumors	6		4		2	
Tumors/Animals	28/33	264±84	29/31	241±84	16/26	224±80

inhibitors showed a significant decrease in total tumors yield, especially among the more frequent kidney tumors.

In summary, we confirmed that hormonal contraceptives do not unquestionably exhibit direct carcinogenic effect. We were also unable to demonstrate a potentiation of a carcinogen in the form of an increased tumor yield or a shortened induction time. Finally, our experiments indicate that treatment with hormonal contraceptives induces no shift in the organotropic effect of a carcinogen with a broad spectrum of organ tumors.

Summary

Wistar rats were treated on three successive days with 40 mg nitrosomethylurea/kg body weight/animal/day. One experimental group received an aqueous suspension of an oral contraceptive (2,5 LYNDIOL®) over a period of thirty days, prior to treatment with carcinogen; a second experimental group was treated with oral contraceptives over a period of thirty days, following carcinogen treatment. No significant differences were observed in a statistical evaluation of the induced tumors. The only demonstrated difference was that rats pretreated with oral contraceptives showed a significant decrease in tumor yield, especially among nephroblastomas.

References

Dallenbach-Hellweg, G.: Endometrium. Berlin-Heidelberg-New York: Springer 1969.

Druckrey, H., Preussmann, R., Ivankovic, S., Schmähl, D.: Z. Krebsforsch. **69**, 103 (1967).

Geschickter, C. F., Hartmann, C. G.: Cancer (Philad.) **12**, 767 (1959).

Gordan, G. S.: Int. Congr. Series 112, Excerpta med. (Amst.) 1961.

Hillemanns, H. G.: Hormonale Kontrazeptiva. Aktuelle Probleme aus dem Gebiet der Cancerologie III. 3. Heidelberger Symposion. H. Lettré und G. Wagner. Berlin-Heidelberg-New York: Springer 1971.

Ober, W. B.: J. clin. Path. **19**, 138 (1966).

Pincus, G.: Modern trends in endocrinology. 2nd. series. Ed.: H. Gardiner-Hill. New York: P. B. Hoeber 1961.

Stern, E., Mickey, M. R.: Brit. J. Cancer **23**, 391 (1969).

Thomas, C., Schmähl, D.: Z. Krebsforsch. **66**, 125 (1964).

Thomas, C., Bollmann, R.: Experientia (Basel) **25**, 50 (1969).

Thomas, C., So, B. T.: Arzneimittelforsch. **19**, 1077 (1969).

Wallach, S., Hennemann, P. H.: J. Amer. med. Ass. **171**, 1637 (1959).

Wilson, R. A.: J. Amer. med. Ass. **182**, 327 (1962).

Role of Regional Lymph Nodes in Growth and Metastasis Formation of Methylcholanthrene-induced Sarcomas of Golden Hamsters*

P. STRÄULI and R. LINDENMANN

Introduction

The role of regional lymph nodes (RLN) in growth and spread of cancer is a matter of considerable controversy. For a long period, the debate centered on the problem of tumor containment in RLN. On the one hand, it was known that RLN can act as temporary barriers against tumor spread. On the other hand, it was experienced in innumerable instances that after collapse of the barrier function, RLN appear as a particularly fertile soil for tumor growth. As an issue from this ambiguity, surgical oncology became accustomed to the rule that RLN should be removed together with the primary tumor. Today, this established standard is challenged by many immunologists. There is an increasing tendency to assume that on principle, all malignant tumors have specific antigens. On this basis, it is argued that immune reactions elicited by these antigens are first localized in RLN which, therefore, should be retained unless grossly involved by tumor growth. Thus, an influence on premetastatic tumor development and not only on dissemination is ascribed to RLN. There are, however, two a priori objections to the claim of RLN retainment. First, immune reactions in these nodes do not necessarily favor the host, and secondly, reactions once started in RLN sooner or later spread to other parts of the lymphoreticular system. The transition from regional to general sensitization can hardly be estimated under clinical conditions. In experimental research, the suggestion is near at hand to compare tumor development in the presence and in the absence of RLN. The first investigation of this kind which has come to our knowledge dates from 1937 (AULER and SCHILLING). In this study as well as in a series of later investigations, transplantable tumors were used. The disadvantage of this model, even in a syngeneic system, is its dissimilarity with the natural course of the host-tumor encounter. In the latter, RLN gradually acquire a series of morphological alterations which influence the mechanical and biological aspects of the barrier function (STRÄULI). Contrarily, transplanted tumors of sufficient malignancy rapidly invade RLN of "text book structure", i. e. unadapted to the presence of a tumor in the tributary area. It stands to reason that only autochthonous tumors with strong antigenicity elicit obvious reactions in the draining nodes. We have used

* This research was supported by a grant-in-aid from the Krebsliga des Kantons Zürich.

methylcholanthrene (MC)-induced sarcomas for which the existence of distinct tumor-specific antigens has frequently been demonstrated since the original description by PREHN and MAIN in 1957. To study the role of RLN in local growth and metastasis formation of such tumors, we compared the two parameters in non-operated animals and in animals in which the RLN (and to a certain extent the corresponding contralateral nodes [CLN] and the spleen) had been removed prior to MC application.

Material and Methods

Induction of Tumors

Two-month-old non-inbred golden hamsters of both sexes received 1 mg 20-methylcholanthrene in 0.1 ml olive oil by s. c. injection in the right flank. Control animals received 0.1 ml olive oil alone.

Control of Tumor Growth

At weekly intervals, the individual tumors were compared with calibrated spheres of plasticine. In this way, the time required to attain the following, arbitrarily determined, sizes was registered for each tumor:

Phase 1 0—3 mm diameter
Phase 2 3—20 mm diameter
Phase 3 20—30 mm diameter

Determination of RLN Topography

India ink was injected s. c. into the right flank. If the site of injection corresponded to that of MC in the main experimental group, the two axillary lymph nodes
lymphonodus axillaris proprius (Ln. ax. prop.)
lymphonodus axillaris accessorius (Ln. ax. ac.)
of the injection side were regularly stained after 1—3 hours. If the injection was made near the inguinal region, the inguinal node
lymphonodus inguinalis (Ln. ing.)
was stained instead of or together with the axillary nodes. With respect to the possibility of tumor growth in a caudal direction, the inguinal node was included in our definition of RLN.

Extirpation of RLN (CLN, Spleen)

Extirpations were performed under general anesthesia 2—3 days before MC injection. The ablative procedures were:

RLN (main experiments)
RLN + CLN
Spleen
RLN + spleen

Results

Fibrosarcomas in various degrees of differentiation developed in nearly 100% of a total of 150 hamsters treated with MC. In occasional large tumors the overlying skin was ulcerated, and/or the center was necrotic. These tumors were excluded from the evaluation.

Local Growth

Table 1 demonstrates the mean duration of the three phases of tumor growth in non-operated female and male hamsters. In males the three phases are longer, but only in phase 1 is the difference significant. As the same animals could be followed through phase 1 and phase 2, the sums of the two phases in females and in males can be statistically evaluated; again the difference in significant. Fig. 1 (upper part) shows that it is not only the mean duration of phase 1 and phase 2 which differs in female and male animals. The distribution of individual growth periods up to the 20 mm size is different too, shorter periods being more frequent in females and longer ones in males.

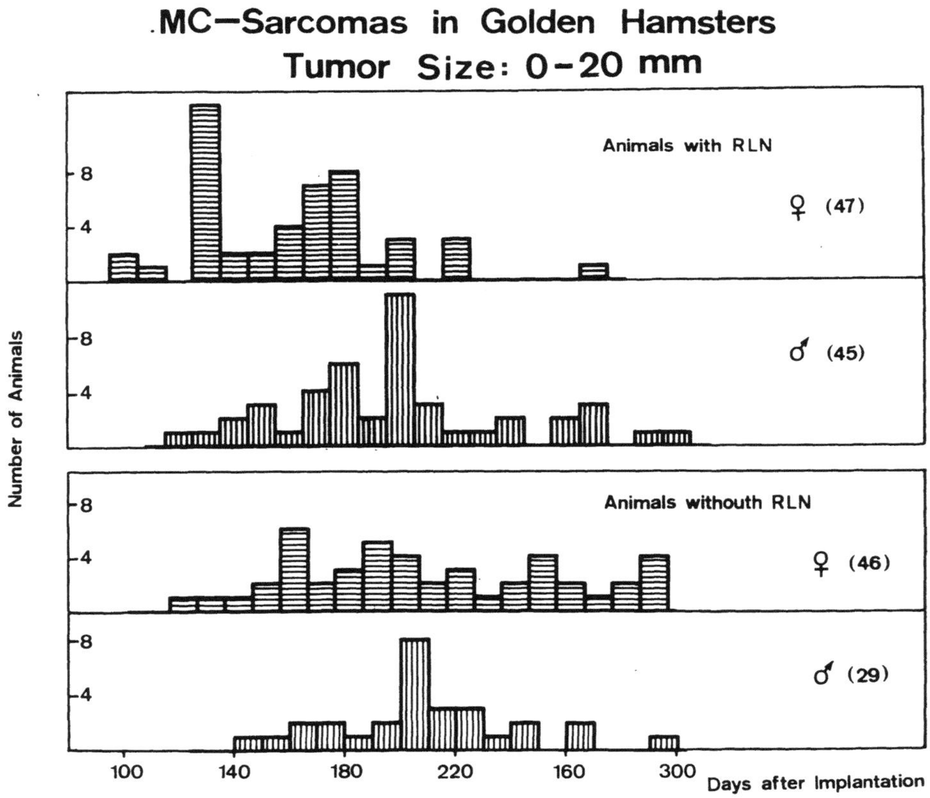

Fig. 1.

Table 1. Tumor development in animals with regional lymph nodes

Phase	Mean duration in days		P
	♀	♂	
1	104 (40)	136 (39)	< 0.003
2	65 (40)	76 (39)	0.11
3	13 (25)	15 (22)	0.08
1+2	169 (40)	212 (39)	< 0.003

( ) Number of animals.

After extirpation of the RLN, the sex difference in tumor development is abolished. This is due to a prolongation of the mean duration of phase 1 and phase 2 in females. As Fig. 1 (lower part) demonstrates, the distribution of individual growth periods in the two sexes is equal and corresponds to tumor development in non-operated male animals.

A comparison of the data for both sexes (Table 2) with those for male animals in Table 1 shows the lack of significant differences. Table 2 further indicates that removal of RLN alone or together with CLN has the same effect.

Extirpation of the spleen has the same effect as removal of RLN. Combined extirpation, RLN + spleen, does not increase the effect of the single procedures.

Table 2. Tumor development in animals without regional lymph nodes (RLN) and without regional and contralateral lymph nodes (RLN + CLN)

Phase	Mean duration in days			
	Without RLN		Without RLN + CLN	
	♀	♂	♀	♂
1	163 (32)	148 (19)	149 (18)	140 (11)
2	65 (30)	63 (18)	63 (18)	69 (11)
3	14 (27)	16 (18)	15 (18)	16 (10)

( ) Number of Animals.

Metastasis Formation

With very few exceptions only animals with sarcomas of more than 30 mm size developed metastases, both of lymphogenous and hematogenous origin.

The frequency of metastases in RLN of non-operated animals is indicated in Table 3. In the same group of animals, lung metastases were found in 50% and kidney metastases in 2%.

Table 4 shows the situation after ablative procedures. A significant increase of hematogenous spread became apparent after removal of RLN, a still larger one

Table 3. Metastases in regional lymph nodes in animals with tumors of > 30 mm

Lymphonodus axillaris proprius	22 = 38%
Lymphonodus axillaris accessorius	8 = 14%
Lymphonodus inguinalis	5 = 9%
Total number of animals	58 = 100%
No sex difference in frequency and pattern	

Table 4. Formation of hematogenous metastases in animals with tumors of > 30 mm

Ablative procedure	No. of animals	Percentage of animals with metastases in Lungs	Kidney	Heart
None	58	50	2	—
RLN removed	52	62	10	4
RLN + CLN removed	33	76	9	—
Spleen removed	24	50	4	—
RLN + spleen removed	30	83	13	3

after removal of both RLN and CLN. Extirpation of the spleen had no effect, but lack of RLN and spleen raised the frequency of metastases to the highest level observed.

Discussion

Our most intriguing observation is the retarding effect of the lack of RLN or spleen on tumor development in female hamsters. The facilitation of early tumor growth in non-operated female animals cannot be conclusively explained at the moment. It appears to be in contrast to the "immunological superiority of the femal" (GRAFF *et al.*) which is a well-established fact in mice. In this species, a higher readiness of females to resistance against MC-sarcomas was demonstrated both in syngeneic transplantation experiments (BLOOM and HILDEMANN) and in autochthonous induction (MARCHANT). As in several other aspects, the hamster may react unlike the mouse. However, there remains the possibility that female hamsters, in accordance with an immunological superiority, react earlier than male animals, but that this lead results in enhancement. As a mass of tumor cells too small to form a palpable take is nevertheless sufficient to induce local or even systemic sensitization (HAMMOND *et al.*), it may be argued that a factor released from RLN and/or spleen during an early phase of tumor development enhances growth of the tumor. Eventually a particular condition of the tumor bed (corium and subcutis) in female animals, as it was recently described for mice by MUNZINGER and GOERTTLER, is a co-factor of this mechanism.

In the course of the present investigation, lymph nodes and spleens were examined histologically. As the results contribute very little to an understanding of the first phase of tumor development, they will be presented in a separate publication and in a more general context. None the less, a few points should be mentioned here.

Morphological changes in RLN, as compared to CLN, were only tangible in animals with tumors that had reached the 3 mm size, and in most animals, unequivocal differences were only found in animals with tumors larger than 20 mm. Alterations consisted in

— increase in weight

— increased number of germinal centers with increased number of mitotic cells in these centers

— increased number of cells labeled with 3H-thymidine in germinal centers, paracortical area and medulla

— increased number of immunoglobulin-containing (= immunofluorescent) cells in the medulla.

It was examined whether these alterations appear in non-regional nodes after extirpation of the RLN. We were unable to find them in the submental nodes (lymphocentrum submentale) and in CLN of sarcoma-bearing hamsters without RLN. However, an obvious increase in weight and in the number of plasma cells was registered in these nodes if large tumors had developed in animals without RLN + spleen. This indicates a compensation of the considerable loss of lymphoreticular tissue, at least with regard to plasma cell production.

According to these morphological findings, RLN are the seat of proliferation involving T and B lymphocytes. Cell-bound and humoral immune reactions can thus be assumed for the period of the established tumor. Due to the coarseness of the morphological methods employed, the beginning of these mechanisms cannot be traced back to an early stage of tumor development. We can only say that these reactions — which must begin some time after MC application — are unable to prevent the local growth of sarcomas. This does not exclude temporarily retarding or accelerating effects on tumor growth. As acceleration could be abolished by removal of the spleen as well as by removal of the RLN, it cannot represent an exclusively regional effect.

In animals with RLN metastases, tumor foci were sometimes found to be surrounded by proliferating lymph node cells. Whatever the time sequence of metastatic growth and lymph node reactions, the latter do not seem to have a definitive, locally damaging effect on tumor cells. Such an effect might be exerted, however, on tumor cells on the way in lymph and blood. At any rate, spread of MC-sarcomas, contrarily to local growth, is not a 100% event. Whether this has anything to do with defense reactions remains an open question. The increased frequency of distant metastases after extirpation of the RLN must be partly attributed to the lack of the barrier function. However, the additional increase of spread after removal of RLN + spleen favors the argument that distant sectors of the lymphoreticular system contribute to the control of metastases.

Several recent experimental investigations with carcinogen-induced tumors transplanted in syngeneic hosts have demonstrated that presence or absence of RLN has no discernible effect on local growth and spread (Bard *et al.*, 1965; Bard *et al.*, 1969; Hammond and Rolley). The results of the present study are in general agreement with these previous findings. Yet they do not justify the statement that there is no functional difference at all between regional and non-regional nodes. In accordance with experiences in allogeneic transplantation models, RLN can be assumed to operate, during a short period of tumor development, as the only site of specific immunological manifestations. Extension of sensitization to other parts of the lymphoreticular system and particularly its largest organ, the spleen, occurs early. In transplantation experiments, cells from RLN as well as from the spleen can be used for adoptive transfer of immunity to chemically induced tumors, although the same cells within their original host are unable to interfere with the growth of the tumor transplant (RLN: Bard *et al.*, 1965; Bard *et al.*, 1969; spleen: Fisher and Hammond; Bard *et al.*, 1969). In spite of the rapid generalization of immunological reactivity, the RLN remain the sector of the lymphoreticular system most heavily and continuously bombarded by tumor antigen (at least before the establishment of metastases). Alexander *et al.* (1969; 1970) have demonstrated that this exposition of RLN can result in a failure to release sensitized lymphocytes (immunoblasts). As distal nodes respond normally to the presence of the tumor, this functional impairment is strictly local. The observation of Alexander *et al.* points to a special situation which distinguishes RLN from all other lymphoreticular organs. And yet this does not imply that RLN are irreplaceable. According to all available evidence, their function is very smoothly taken over by other parts of the system. Theoretically, this compensation requires the intactness of the afferent limb of immunological reactivity, a condition which apparently is never queried in experimental practice.

There is no generally acceptable answer to the crucial question of surgical oncology whether RLN favor the host or the tumor. All depends on the sequence of events in the host-tumor-system. Without doubt RLN are a topographically privileged site of metastasis formation. On the other hand, there is a period in which they represent the specific site of immunological manifestations. The duration of this period is ill-defined, and in the stage of the clinically detectable tumor, it is very likely that sensitization has long ago become a generalized phenomenon. There is, however, the challenging observation of Alexander *et al.* that after removal of the primary tumor, RLN rapidly release the immunoblasts accumulated during the period of immune paralysis. The effect of this event on metastases requires further investigation. The basic problem concerns the applicability of such models to an understanding of the natural course of human cancer. The gap between tumor immunology in experimental animals and human beings is still large. As has recently been demonstrated by Griffiths (1970), it might be bridged by carefully selected studies in human cancer patients.

Summary

Local growth of fibrosarcomas occurred in practically 100% of golden hamsters after a single s.c. injection of 1 mg methylcholanthrene. Up to a size of 20 mm, tumor development took a more rapid course in female than in male animals. Further growth did not show a significant difference between the sexes. Removal of the regional lymph nodes or the spleen before methylcholanthrene application suppressed the rapidly growing tumors, i. e. those occurring predominantely in females. Thus the ablative procedures resulted in equalization of tumor development in the two sexes. — Metastasis formation was an irregular event and only observed in animals with tumors of at least 30 mm size. Extirpation of the regional lymph nodes was not followed by spread to other (non-regional) nodes. It intensified, however, the formation of lung metastases. No such effect was observed after removal of the spleen, whereas extirpation of both the draining nodes and the spleen had a highly promoting effect on hematogenous spread.

These results are compatible with the following interpretation of the significance of the regional lymph nodes: Only for a short period during tumor development are they the specific site of immunological manifestations which eventually result in tumor enhancement; later, and at any rate in the phase of the clinically detectable tumor, sensitization is a generalized phenomenon in the lymphoreticular system, and the role of the draining nodes is restricted to their local barrier function.

References

ALEXANDER, P., BENSTED, J., DELORME, E. J., HALL, J. G., HODGETT, J.: Proc. roy. Soc. **174 B**, 237 (1968).

ALEXANDER, P., HALL, J. G.: Advanc. Cancer Res. **13**, 1 (1970).

AULER, H., SCHILLING, W.: Z. Krebsforsch. **46**, 241 (1937).

BARD, D. S., HAMMOND, W. G., KETCHAM, A. S.: Surg. Forum **16**, 110 (1965).

BARD, D. S., HAMMOND, W. G., PILCH, Y. H.: Cancer Res. **29**, 1379 (1969).

BARD, D. S., HAMMOND, W. G., KETCHAM, A. S.: Cancer Res. **29**, 1125 (1969).

BLOOM, EDA T., HILDEMANN, W. H.: Transplant. Bull. **10**, 321 (1970).

FISHER, J. C., HAMMOND, W. H.: Surg. Forum **17**, 102 (1966).

GRIFFITHS, C. O.: Trans. Amer. Acad. Ophthal. Otolaryng. **74**, 291 (1970).

GRAFF, R. J., LAPPE, M. A., SNELL, G. D.: Transplant. Bull. **7**, 105 (1969).

HAMMOND, W. G., FISHER, J. C., ROLLEY, R. T.: Surgery **62**, 124 (1967).

HAMMOND, W. G., ROLLEY, R. T.: Cancer (Philad.) **25**, 368 (1970).

MARCHANT, JUNE: Brit. J. Cancer **23**, 377 (1969).

MUNZINGER, H., GOERTTLER, K.: Z. Krebsforsch. **73**, 342 (1970).

PREHN, R. T., MAIN, J. M.: J. nat. Cancer Inst. **18**, 769 (1957).

STRÄULI, P.: In: Surgical Oncology. Eds.: F. SAEGESSER and J. PETTAVEL. Bern-Stuttgart-Vienna: Huber 1970, pp. 161—176.

Subject Index

*43 Nomenclature, Methodology and Results of Clinical Trials in Acute Leukemias (Symposium). Edited by G. MATHÉ, L. SCHWARZENBERG, P. POUILLART, Villejuif. Cloth DM 58,—; US $ 22.40

*44 Special Topics in Carcinogenesis (Symposium). Edited by E. GRUNDMANN, Münster. Cloth DM 58,—; US $ 22.40

Special Supplement: Biology of Amphibian Tumors. Edited by M. MIZELL, New Orleans. Cloth DM 86,—; US $ 33.20

In Production

45 KOLDOVSKY, P., Philadelphia: Carcinoembryonic Antigens

46 MUSSHOFF, K., Freiburg: Diagnosis and Therapy of Malignant Lymphoma

47 MATHÉ, G., WEINER, R., Villejuif: Investigation and Stimulation of Immunity in Cancer Patients (Symposium)

In Preparation

BOIRON, M.: The Viruses of the Leukemia-Sarcoma Complex

CAVALIERE, R., ROSSI-FANELLI, A., MONDOVI, B., and MORICCA, G.: Selective Heat Sensitivity of Cancer Cells

CONNORS, T. A., ROBERTS, J.: Platinum Coordination Complexes in Cancer Chemotherapy (Symposium)

GARATTINI, S., FRANCHI, G.: Chemotherapy of Cancer Dissemination: Methods and Results

GRUNDMANN, E.: Morphology and Cytochemistry of Carcinogenesis

KESSLER, I., AURELIAN, L.: Cancer of the Cervix: Problem, Progress, Prospects

LEVIN, A.: Human Tumour Immunology for Clinicians and Experimentalists

MATHÉ, G.: Immunotherapy of Cancer

MERKOW, L., SLIFKIN, M.: Oncogenic Simian Adenoviruses

OETTGEN, H. F.: Tumor Immunology

RICHTERS, A., SHERWIN, R.: Autochthonous Lymphocyte Interactions with Neoplastic and Non-neoplastic Human Cells

WEIL, R.: Biological and Structural Properties of Polyoma Virus and its DNA

MIX
Papier aus verantwortungsvollen Quellen
Paper from responsible sources
FSC® C105338

If you have any concerns about our products,
you can contact us on
ProductSafety@springernature.com

In case Publisher is established outside the EU,
the EU authorized representative is:
Springer Nature Customer Service Center GmbH
Europaplatz 3, 69115 Heidelberg, Germany

Printed by Libri Plureos GmbH
in Hamburg, Germany